Praise for UPSTAIRS IN THE CRAZY HOUSE

"It is not very often we get to applaud a valiant act. This book is such an act and its author deserves a standing ovation."
—Timothy Findley

"Pick a superlative. 'Brilliant' will do. So will 'original.' . . . deserves all the prized adjectives that hail the best books."
— *Toronto Star*

"Powerful and lyrical, drenched in observation and perfect pitch dialogue. Her own life experience is full of agony and triumph, and her writing resonates with the wisdom and wry humour that comes from self-growth achieved by climbing with the aid of fingernails. It also shines with the splendor of her deeply spiritual self."
—June Callwood

"Pat sees with wonder and understanding, and writes beautifully."
—Joey Slinger

"Capponi's offering is a true and beautiful gift."
— *The Gazette* (Montreal)

"Eloquent, compassionate, funny, courageous."
—Jane Rule

"A story to make you weep... in this book, which must have taken exceptional courage to write, Capponi, and the light she lets in, shines."
— *The Globe and Mail*

ALSO BY PAT CAPPONI

Bound by Duty: Walking the Beat with Canada's Cops

The War at Home: An Intimate Portrait of Canada's Poor

Dispatches from the Poverty Line

Upstairs in the Crazy House: The Life of a Psychiatric Survivor

PENGUIN CANADA

BEYOND THE CRAZY HOUSE

Pat Capponi is the author of the critically acclaimed memoir *Upstairs in the Crazy House*, as well as *Dispatches from the Poverty Line*, *The War at Home*, and *Bound by Duty*. Capponi has served on numerous agency and hospital boards, developed a Leadership Facilitation program specific to the psychiatric survivor community, and is a founding member of the Gerstein Centre in Toronto. She has been awarded the Order of Ontario and the C.M. Hincks award from the Canadian Mental Health Association. She lives in Toronto.

Beyond the Crazy House

Changing the Future of Madness

PAT CAPPONI

PENGUIN
CANADA

PENGUIN CANADA

Published by the Penguin Group

Penguin Books, a division of Pearson Canada, 10 Alcorn Avenue, Toronto, Ontario,
  Canada M4V 3B2
Penguin Books Ltd, 80 Strand, London WC2R 0RL, England
Penguin Putnam Inc., 375 Hudson Street, New York, New York 10014, U.S.A.
Penguin Books Australia Ltd, 250 Camberwell Road, Camberwell, Victoria 3124, Australia
Penguin Books India (P) Ltd, 11, Community Centre, Panchsheel Park,
  New Delhi – 110 017, India
Penguin Books (NZ) Ltd, cnr Rosedale and Airborne Roads, Albany, Auckland 1310,
  New Zealand
Penguin Books (South Africa) (Pty) Ltd, 24 Sturdee Avenue, Rosebank 2196, South Africa

Penguin Books Ltd, Registered Offices: 80 Strand, London WC2R 0RL, England

First published 2003

10 9 8 7 6 5 4 3 2 1

Copyright © Pat Capponi, 2003

Manufactured in Canada.

NATIONAL LIBRARY OF CANADA CATALOGUING IN PUBLICATION

Capponi, Pat, 1949–
   Beyond the crazy house : changing the future of madness / Pat Capponi.

ISBN 0-14-100510-6

1. Mentally ill—Biography. 2. Mental illness. I. Title.

RC464.A1C36   2003   616.89'0092   C2002-905894-5

Visit Penguin Books' website at **www.penguin.ca**

Contents

Acknowledgements

To all those, present and past, who lent their support:

Paul Quinn, Reva Gerstein, Elizabeth Gray, June Callwood, Nora McCabe, Joey Slinger,

Ernest Hirschbach, Diana and Julia Capponi, Pauline Pariser, Donald Bennett, Becky McFarlane, and the folks at the Raging Spoon, Away Express, the Out of this World Café, and the Ontario Council of Alternative Business.

Special thanks to my friend and publisher, Cynthia Good, and heartfelt thanks to editor Susan Folkins and my agent Bev Slopen.

And there are no words to express my appreciation to those who dared to contribute their stories.

Foreword
by Reva Gerstein

I had the good fortune to become acquainted with Pat Capponi nearly 20 years ago. I had been invited by the mayor of Toronto to chair a task force to develop a comprehensive master plan for the city to implement the new policy of deinstitutionalizing psychiatric patients.

My background and experience in the mental health field dates back to Professor William Line, my great teacher at the University of Toronto, and Dr. Clarence Hincks, the founder of the mental health movement in Canada and the United States. My life path has taken many twists and turns, and my c.v. includes items such as Founder and past Chair of the Hincks Treatment Centre, Founder and Chair of the Gerstein Crisis Centre; past Chair of The Canadian Institute for Advanced Research, and Chancellor Emeritus of the University of Western Ontario.

My earliest experience in the mental health field was, in many ways, traditional. In the 1950s, Dr. Hincks and I were told of a new medication for mental illness, which would make it possible for psychiatric patients to be treated, with the probability of deinstitutionalization. Many of us within the professional community accepted this medical model. It was Pat Capponi, as a member of my Task Force Advisory Committee, who turned my head around. She convinced me, at numerous public hearings at the City Hall and at smaller meetings with "survivors" throughout the city, of the limitations of relying on medication alone for treatment.

Pat Capponi's *Beyond the Crazy House* is an impressive, remarkable book. In it she explains that "The needs of members of the psychiatric community are not so different, really, from anyone else's needs—a home, a job, a friend." This book is courageous, insightful, painful, penetrating and provocative. Capponi takes us on a journey that is neither for the faint of heart nor for those who would safeguard traditional professional territories. The scope and depth of her deliberations is profound. Her documentation of several personal histories, including her own, will remain deeply etched in my psyche.

Pat Capponi has pointed the way to "Changing the Future of Madness."

Dr. Reva Gerstein
Companion, Order of Canada and
Member of the Order of Ontario
December 2002
Toronto

Introduction

In the early eighties, I stepped out the front door of my boarding home for ex-psychiatric patients in the west end of Toronto, on my way to becoming one of the people that the other residents and I had watched from the verandah—those people who walk freely to and from work or school, or stroll casually from shop to shop. The few clothes and possessions I had were packed inside the ubiquitous green garbage bag that passes for luggage in the poverty-riddled ex-mental patient community. Added to that was my small hoard of dollars, a welfare cheque, a pack of cigarettes, and a fearful, wavering determination to try again. It was like the first time I left home, when I ran away to a hospital ward with nothing in my pockets, or years later, when I escaped my sister's apartment to go to college, fifty dollars between me and the street.

The boarding home was not a place people left for something better. In my four years there, no one had left voluntarily. Evictions were common, abandoning people to the streets, as were recalls to the psychiatric hospital down the road. Who was I to think I could return to the world that had banished us? I was leaving behind seventy men and women, de-institutionalized patients from the Queen Street, Whitby, and Lakeshore Mental Health Centres—isolated, medicated, forgotten people, ravaged by poverty and loss—my friends, my peers, my community. We were modern-day lepers, set apart, kept apart, in dark, crowded rooms infested with mice and lice, while beyond the walls life played out in sunlight and possibilities. Even so, I had felt safe and cared for at the boarding house. With the help of my friends, I had regained some sense of my own strength, some memory of who I was before all this, before I became just another chronic mental patient.

I didn't want to leave.

I had nothing in common anymore with the world out there. I had seen and felt and endured too much simply to pick up where I'd left off, to pretend that I cared about life as it was supposed to be lived, that I'd never seen what is done to those who stumble and fall. There were scars on my arms, my heart, and my soul that had little to do with the diagnosed depressive illness that had set me apart, that had sent me again and again and again to psychiatric wards in search of a cure, until they tired of me and sent me to live with others for whom there was no hope.

Yet, despite the fears and the temptation to stay, I had to go. I had a promise to fulfill and a commitment to undertake.

As I left the boarding house, I knew they were watching me from the dirty windows of the rooms facing King Street—Gary, Miss Pattison, Dennis, Delores, Alice, phony Father Francis, and Haddie—wanting to call me back, to warn me away from this folly. Just as ordinary citizens are frightened of ever stepping inside our madhouse, stepping out into the busy streets where ex-psychiatric patients are so visible and vulnerable to assaults, taunts, and judgments, was truly terrifying for me. I had to relearn the rhythm of walking, of keeping pace with the pedestrian flow. I had to try to keep my head up, instead of focusing on the pavement. I had to lose that sense of a blinking neon sign over my head warning *mental patient, mental patient.* And the chaos was not just inside my head. The traffic, the noise, the light: It was a sensory overload. My new and still so fragile determination seemed to evaporate—I could hardly get air into my lungs—and fits of panic almost drove me screaming back to the safety of the house.

This was madness; leaving was madness. I didn't belong out here; they were right to put me away. I was still broken, broken beyond repair. I should admit that, and return to my third-floor room in the crazy house.

Though many can never bring themselves to take that first step, somehow I kept walking, towards life, not away from it. Then, in 1992, I wrote *Upstairs in the Crazy House,* a book about the people I had come to love in the Parkdale boarding home on King Street West. My experiences living in that house led me to wonder about all the men and women who, over the centuries, had been labelled and confined to cold, grey, mental hospitals out of "care." Were these people victimized by their illnesses or by society's inability to understand their simple craving to be a part of life, to experience love, or even just the warmth of a summer's day?

In our wilful ignorance, we have done, and continue to do, terrible things to "mental patients." Across North America, hospitals have been closed, but governments have refused to re-invest the savings into the communities where the de-institutionalized were sent. We have abandoned people to profit-seeking landlords of boarding and rooming houses, to hostel beds, and to the streets. And in trying to explain why so many ex-psychiatric patients lead such desperate lives, we have continued to blame the illness and not the terrible quality of life many endure, with day-to-day suffering, excruciating poverty, and loss.

There has been a recent movement, however, to change the kind of care offered to de-institutionalized mental patients, from the grim, overcrowded boarding houses to something that is more like real life. I've been privileged to observe and share in this process of renewal and it has been a long, glorious struggle. The battle has gone far beyond the walls that were put up to keep us "safe," watched, medicated, and apart. It has gone beyond welfare and disability cheques, drug cards, and drop-ins, into places where no one expected they would have to deal with mental patients— hospital boardrooms, government committees and task forces, colleges and universities—and onto the country's workforce and tax rolls. In the vanguard of this movement were men and women who had to overcome the challenges of poverty, pain, and pills to believe in their own empowerment first, and then in the potential of their peers. In the face of the public's perception of the mentally ill as incapable, frightening, dangerous people (released from years of institutional "safety" by liberal do-gooders and inflicted on the communities that had excluded them in the first place), these men and women gave a new definition to the term *right to life*.

These survivors are different from the ex-psychiatric patients I lived with in my boarding home. Though they had been admitted to hospitals often, they had not been institutionalized for decade-plus years, a common experience in the house. With more time outside, they could nurture hopes and dreams; they could stay in school (between bouts of illness); they could try different jobs, and they could see how the rest of the world lived. Though their pain was the same, anger had not been wrung out of them through the grey sameness of days; they could resist dependency and unlearn institutional behaviour.

As well, our community of psychiatric survivors was eager to challenge the hugely profitable "non-profit" mental health industry that had grown up around us. Hospitals, unions, charitable foundations, agencies, and pharmaceutical companies had been charged with our care and purported to speak for us. Everyone but us, however, profited from our illnesses, through jobs, status, and power. Into this closed, self-congratulatory system came a reality check from our unexpected quarter—from the ragtag collection of modern-day, feisty Oliver Twists who didn't just say "Please sir, I want some more," but instead demanded the absolute baseline entitlement to a home, a job, and a friend. Although their grasp of reality was suspect at best and required volumes of medication and watchfulness to sustain, they had a fighting chance. In more ways than one, they needed to be crazy to take on a system that saw them only as their diseases.

The needs of members of the psychiatric community are not so different, really, from anyone else's needs—a home, a job, a friend.

When those goals are frustrated and made inaccessible, however, madness can be a response. It took pioneers from our devastated community to challenge the public perception of who we are and what we can achieve when given the smallest opportunity to do so—it took pioneers who are reshaping the face of madness.

Over the years of my journey that began when I walked away from my boarding home determined to make a difference, I met many of the people whose stories are told here. For some, their psychiatric careers were just starting as I was leaving mine behind; others got out shortly after I did. We learned to work around our demons, to diminish their impact, to medicate them back to sleep when necessary, even to return to hospital wards when they got out of our control. None of us was cured. There is no cure.

The challenge for psychiatric survivors, then, is the same for anyone with a chronic illness: learn everything you can about what it is you're supposed to have; don't let it consume you; pay attention to triggers; learn what eases the pain; and understand how frustration and behaviour can sometimes undermine you. There are no guides to follow, no experts to consult. Although the medical-pharmaceutical system knows how to deal with ravening psychic pain, that pain is difficult to categorize (witness the frequency of misdiagnosis), and can only be artificially muted with prescription drugs that are marginally safer than the street drugs and alcohol mental health patients will use to self-medicate. Individual human needs require individual human responses and reassurances, and the medical system is not good at delivering that. The great gap between caregivers and recipients is widening as the "caring society" in which we live continues to devolve into a Darwinian enclosure, casting out those who don't measure up.

An examination of what causes psychiatric disorders (other than those for which pills can be prescribed) threatens society's collective self-image—the majority view of the world as a sane, livable place. Mind you, the events of September 11 left many people reaching for the Prozac. The explosions that took down the twin towers created deep fissures in many lives, exposing fears we didn't have to face before—of anthrax, terrorists, nuclear attacks, and war. World events continue to keep us off-balance and edgy—Israel and the Palestinians, Pakistan and India, the US and Iraq—everyone is posturing, going to the brink, taking the rest of us with them. In North America, our belief in corporations has been badly shaken by senior executives who chose greed over duty. And our faith in religious institutions now seems naive, as more and more victims of abuse come forward to speak the truth.

These are dark times. They are times that even the most paranoid individual couldn't conceive. Such times demand strength, independence, and courage from everyone, if we are to survive. Certainly, if those of us deemed least able to do so have been fully engaged in a constant struggle to rise above our fears and limitations, to break out of our roles as mental patients and into real life, and to bring—whenever possible—our peers along with us, then those less challenged have no excuse for failure.

Here are our stories.

PART ONE

The Roots
of Madness

1.

When Madness Is the Only Rational Response

Children have long been the silent victims of their parents' fighting. Though most never talk about it, witnessing physical abuse at home causes them serious emotional damage, according to a new Statistics Canada study. Such children are more than twice as likely to be physically aggressive themselves and they have much higher rates of depression, worry and frustration than other children.

> —Elaine Carey, "Witnessing Abuse Damages Kids: Study," *Toronto Star*, July 14, 2001

There is a great deal of debate about the origins of mental illness—whether it's a biochemical misfiring, the result of early family experiences, or some lethal combination of both. This debate matters, because if we assume everything is related to physiology then the primary, "sane" response is to treat mental illness with pharmaceuticals—a clean, easy solution, and one we have a lot of comfort with in the twenty-first century. It removes parental guilt and individual responsibility; it pathologizes and medicates behaviours; it elevates a pseudo-science to the big leagues. There is profit in the search for "magic bullets," in the research, development, and marketing of newer, better, and costlier medications for the mind. Ultimately, though, this is a soulless and limiting response to pain and distress, however caused. In the rush to study, dissect, and understand the brain, we've forgotten that the whole individual is greater than the sum of her parts.

Whatever the cause of mental illness, a narrow approach to therapy leads to less effective interventions. We will look at mental illness and its origins in the lives of psychiatric survivors, some of whom had craziness inflicted on them through early abuse, others who—in spite of supportive, loving families— found themselves enduring a sudden, inexplicable onslaught of madness. However people become ill, they are not that illness embodied; they are people first, and they would be best served by assisting their efforts to learn, to grow, and to achieve a measure of quality of life.

Though there may come a time when science will allow an individual, feeling at the end of his or her tether, to walk into a hospital with no human workers, submit to a diagnostic machine that will test brainwaves, skin, blood, and urine in seconds, and then dispense a soothing drug that will slam the door on voices or calm self-destructive urges, we are not there yet. Thank God.

For now, the response to people who, as children, have suffered from feelings of powerlessness and abuse by authority figures, who have felt somewhere deep inside that they've brought all this down on themselves because they weren't good enough or lovable enough, who've never felt safe and wanted, is to put them in a place where they once again have no power, where they are subjected to negative judgments and labels that confirm their fears that it was their own fault. Here the abuse comes packaged as therapy or protection: bubble rooms (solitary confinement in a room with a mattress and a small fishbowl-like viewing window), injections of powerful antipsychotics, and four-point restraints (the arms and legs are tied down at the wrists and ankles).

Laurie Hall and Barry D'Costa are only two out of thousands of survivors who were driven crazy by their home lives. Their search for a cure, a way to escape the feelings planted deep inside during their formative years, is a search many have undertaken, with varying degrees of success.

· · ·

Though I had heard of Laurie Hall, the executive director of Away Express Courier Service, a survivor business, I didn't actually meet her until 1995 when we ran into each other at a hearing into the fate of the Ontario Advocacy Commission held by the newly elected Harris government. In T-shirt and jeans, her bare arms covered with dramatic, self-inflicted scars, Laurie had taken her place in front of the gathered politicians and argued passionately for the commission to continue its necessary work. Her voice was low and smoky, her delivery compelling. Even knowing that the decision had already been made to disband the commission and that the hearing was just window-dressing, she made her points with devastating accuracy.

Months later, when unemployment and excruciating poverty were making me "mental," it was Laurie who said, "Come work with us." Away was, in many ways, her territory, the place that had recognized her potential even before she could see it, had nourished her, and helped her grow from courier to executive director, from mental patient to psychiatric survivor leader.

These days, Laurie is one of the most respected psychiatric survivor leaders in Ontario and the country. She is a bridge-builder and an inspiration to many still trapped within the mental health system. She has fought for a place at the table with bureaucrats and politicians, and for the right to help shape government policies. Though diminutive, and at times shy, she shines like a lighthouse through the deep fog of her community, using humour and her experiences to encourage peers to overcome their "illnesses" and their poverty. But it was a long journey, fraught with danger and self-destruction, to find her strengths.

Laurie's bedroom closet was the safest place in the isolated old brick house her great-grandfather had built. The bedroom itself would not do. She would hear her dad stomping up the steps, and then the door would slam open and there would be no escape. Laurie was the eldest of five children. When she was little, her father treated her like the son he wanted, taking her everywhere. She'd ride the tractor with him on their small farm with its mix of beef cattle, a milk cow, a few pigs, and a vegetable plot. When he became apprenticed to a mechanic, she went with him to the garage, learning the names of the tools and the parts. She was six when her brother Scott was born, and soon after she was left behind with the women at the house to do girl things, while Scott was taken along with her dad. The rejection left her angry and confused. Later, she remembers her dad bought yet another second-hand pick-up truck, one with less rust and fewer dents. He painted a sign on it—S. Hall and Son—as though the rest of them just didn't exist.

Her father, 5'7" and 220 pounds, was short-tempered and abusive; he wouldn't tolerate no for an answer. He had to control everyone and everything, and couldn't hold a job where he had to take orders. So he was at home a lot. Consequently, they didn't have much money—second-hand clothes from cousins were the norm.

He picked on her mother all the time. Laurie especially hated the way he caused her mother to break into helpless tears. Both Laurie and her mom were short and compact, with black hair and brown eyes. Her father had always reserved his physical violence for his eldest daughter, who so closely resembled his wife in every aspect but temperament. Often Laurie tried to get her mother to fight back, suggesting that she pack her bags and escape to something better. Sometimes she almost believed that her mom would find the courage, but she never did.

But Laurie could and would.

On Laurie's last day at home, when she was fifteen, the family gathered around the scarred wooden table in the kitchen, eating lunch and getting ready to go to the town fair. The five children clamoured for their allowances; Laurie's dad demanded to know what they'd done to earn it. The girls, including Laurie, talked about helping their mom in the house, cooking, baking, and cleaning.

"That's not real work, that's woman's work," he shot back, turning to his son to ask what he'd done for his money. Scott had worked in the barn and the fields, and fed the animals—this was manly work, so he got his allowance.

Laurie challenged her dad, saying, "That's not fair."

Her dad swung at her face with his closed fist, knocking her to the floor, while her mother and the rest of the kids ran out to the car as they always did when he went off on Laurie.

"You don't like it, you know what you can do!" he shouted.

This time, the last of many times, she wanted him to be more specific, to actually say that if she didn't like it, she could get the hell out. A good friend of hers had run away a few weeks before, and Children's Aid (CAS) had placed him in a foster home.

"I found that so exciting, the idea that you could get out. That day, we all drove to the fair as though nothing had happened. I met up with my friends, and arranged to go home with one of them."

Just once, she had tried to talk about the hell at home. It had been during a grade seven health class, where the girls were separated from the boys. They'd been talking about spankings and punishments, and the kids said things like, "My dad keeps a strap on the back of the door."

"I had had a particularly bad beating the night before. He'd used horsehair ropes that left large welts on my arms and legs, and I started talking about it. But I didn't get very far before I looked at the faces around me, at the shock on the faces of my classmates, and three things went through my mind very quickly. Number one was: Shut Up. Number two was: they're not talking about the same thing. And the last was: how horrible I must be for my father to be doing this to me. It was my first indication that this wasn't happening to my friends, or to any of the other people that I knew. The teacher never pursued it. In retrospect, I might have been testing the waters, telling myself: Let's put a little out there and see the response. I never talked about it at school again, or anywhere outside of home."

The family that took her in was quite poor. Their house was a ramshackle, falling-down affair, but they had forty acres of vegetable plots that had to be worked, so there were always kids around. Her father came looking for her and told her to get in the truck, saying that he just wanted to talk. Since she'd left her clothes behind, she went back with him to pick them up, telling her friends to come get her if she didn't return in thirty minutes.

He didn't hit her, but he yelled a lot. "How will it look to the neighbours?" he raged. It was especially galling that she'd prefer hardscrabble poverty with the foster family to living at home. What would people think? What lies are you telling about me?

But she was out from under his fist. She packed her clothes, and she was gone.

In spite of the upheaval in her small world, Laurie kept going to classes from her new home—except when all hands were needed in the fields—knowing she wanted an education, wanted a real life.

One day, her mother showed up at her school to speak with each of her teachers: she cried, wrung her hands, and wondered aloud how and why such a thing could happen. Everything was fine at home, could Laurie be on drugs? When class started, Laurie was forced to listen to a rant about respect and filial duty to parents.

"All of a sudden, my teachers couldn't stand me. They totally bought that it was just me being bad. My parents had always been able to pull off the 'stable family' image, and I was threatening it."

Years later, her mother told her in self-defence, "Your father and I always believed in corporal punishment, we didn't mean to hurt you."

She thought she was free, she thought she'd escaped and left behind all the violence, all the pain, succumbing to that brief and common delusion that we can put our past safely behind us and move on.

Given such a shaky start, it's not surprising that Laurie ran into a world of trouble. She moved to Guelph to stay with a friend, and to finish up grade thirteen. She hung out with college students who were through school for the year. Soon everyone had gone back home or away to work, including her roommate. It was hard to come up with the money for rent all on her own, but she found a job that paid minimum wage at a local convenience store. Her hours were from 4 p.m. to 12 midnight. She could easily do her homework there, especially since no one ever came in after 10 p.m.

She could also drink, and this drowned her inhibitions and tapped into her anger, though finding the money to pay for it was challenging. Laurie started to not ring in sales of cartons of cigarettes, just pocketing the money, in the era before cameras and lie-detector tests. Her take began to add up, and the owner had noticed enough to keep tabs on two male employees who were his first suspects, even spying on them. One of the employees was dealing drugs out of the store; but it was Laurie who was responsible for the diminishing inventory. She felt things were closing in on her, and one night, burning with liquid courage from the forty-ouncer she kept hidden in the backroom, she made a plan. She emptied the cash register, stashed the money in a sack, and hid it in the same place as her bottle. Satisfied she was being clever, she then called the cops to report a robbery. (In her less-than-astute state, she figured she could use the money to gradually replace the missing inventory so that they wouldn't be able to tell she'd been stealing.)

The cops were clearly suspicious.

They looked around, and asked if the robber had used a weapon. Laurie said the robber had his hand in his pocket, and something hard was pointing out at her. Could she describe him? In the most general terms possible, she did. The two detectives told her they'd come by her apartment Monday (it was a Friday night) with a sketch artist. It was the longest weekend of her life, and she was very alone, very scared. The conflict between wanting to be stopped and the fear of being caught played out feverishly. When the cops arrived Monday morning, they were not carrying a sketchbook. Casually, they told her about the last case they'd worked where a guy had reported a robbery, but it had turned out he'd stolen the money himself.

She broke.

"I know you know I did it. I just want to confess and give the money back."

They were very sweet to her, these burly plainclothes officers. On the drive to the store to pick up the cash, one of them slipped her a business card, and said, "He's a good lawyer, and he takes legal aid cases." The other cop expressed his regret that it wasn't the owner who'd done the theft, letting Laurie know that they'd had their eyes on the place for a long time. If Laurie came back in a couple of years, he'd be glad to tell her all about it.

It could have been a lot worse; they only charged her with public mischief. She was fingerprinted and photographed, and released with a court date.

She missed it.

The police picked her up at school. Her lawyer showed up at the station, and she didn't have to spend time in the cells. The judge asked for a pre-sentence report, giving the caseworker a month to write it. When it was finished, Laurie found it instructive to read about how she was viewed at school (depressed, withdrawn, doesn't interact with others), how her life looked on paper.

She was given a year's probation, and a probation officer whom she really liked. He would tell her: Laurie, all day I have to deal with rapists and murderers, and then you come in and brighten my world. Many people feel that way about her.

That was in June. By September she had run away from the psychiatric ward where she was enduring her second admission (her first had been the result of an overdose of two bottles of Tylenol). Four days before, she had piled up a bunch of sheets in the linen room and set fire to them. It was a contained fire in a room that would not allow it to spread, but the smoke was so thick the fire department had to bring huge fans to clear it out. No one suspected Laurie, and she was getting very frustrated: What does it take to get caught?

It was dark and cold. Escaping the hospital had been pretty easy, going back to the same store she'd broken into a few times before seemed the thing to do. Not that she thought about it much, she was mostly on automatic pilot, and had been for some time. This night, however, there was a security guard inside the building. He'd left his car running, and the doors open. The backyard of the store was essentially a gravel dump, with artificial hills piled up around the parking lot. She got in the car, slammed the doors shut, and tried to drive up those hills. The car stalled halfway up the second one, and she abandoned it, running away through the night. She returned to the scene a couple of hours later, saw the guard looking up and down the street, and brazenly approached him.

"Are you looking for something?" she asked innocently.

He was angry that someone had stolen his car, but he didn't suspect her. She'd been trying to get caught for some time, and it was a lot harder than she'd thought.

"What does a person have to do?" she muttered to herself.

For months now, under cover of darkness and fuelled by wine or whisky, she'd been "marauding" in the neighbourhood—petty pilfering, breaking windows, removing bikes from backyard sheds and abandoning them a few blocks away. If she was considered so bad and different, then she would act the part. A gradual escalation drew her in deeper.

"At seventeen, I was just this package of compressed rage walking around."

Laurie was already on a year's probation and if she were caught, she'd have to do the time for the first offence, along with whatever she was given for the second conviction. A nurse she liked, whom she'd told just a little about her illegal activity, talked to her. Laurie said she was "really good, one of the few." The floodgates broke and Laurie confessed again. She was never charged and never went to court. Although two police officers were called in, they didn't believe she'd set the fire.

"They were so nice, I think they thought I was really mental."

Laurie was lucky, at least compared with many who now languish in prisons, having finally found ways to make the world pay attention. Living under the thumb of a petty tyrant for years and suffering physical and emotional abuse had left her with a blinding, consuming rage that medications or psychiatric labels could not cover up.

Like Laurie, we don't understand what drives us, but in brief flashes of clarity, we know that we're out of control. We need practical help to validate and then rein in that anger, and we need reassurance that it isn't our fault, that we're not as bad as we fear we are. Unfortunately, that support is often not forthcoming from hospital staff concerned with the smooth operation of the ward, and we're left feeling that we've simply traded one form of abuse for another.

We do know, however, the consequences of trusting, of asking for anything—of setting ourselves up to be hurt, disappointed, or ridiculed. So, again like Laurie, we wrap the ragged remnants of our self-respect around us and hide behind our defiance, declaring our awareness of the reality of indifference or worse lurking behind professions of concern.

*   *   *

Barry D'Costa is a passionate, sensitive, young man, brown-skinned, with finely draw features and expressive eyes. His parents were born in Kenya and their parents in Portuguese Goa.

Barry spent the first six years of his life three hours north of London, England, in an area called the Midlands, and then his parents immigrated to Canada and settled in Kitchener-Waterloo.

Barry read my first book, *Upstairs in the Crazy House*, while living and working in Kitchener-Waterloo, between hospital admissions. It struck a resonant chord in him, and he eventually made his way to Toronto to take up a position with PERC (Parkdale Economic Resources Committee), a fledgling survivor business based at the Parkdale Activity and Recreation Centre. He was part of a leadership group I conducted for the Ontario Council of Alternative Businesses (OCAB); his energy, commitment, and passion made him the best of the best.

Barry grew up watching his mother take constant verbal and physical abuse. There was so much unhappiness, violence, and turmoil in his home that as a child he found it impossible to concentrate at school, or even to stop crying. Teachers may have asked him what was the matter—he doesn't remember—but he wouldn't have, couldn't have, told them anyway.

Fights at home were about anything and everything. He was fourteen when his new baby sister came home from the hospital. He remembers the awe he felt holding her, and the need he had to protect her, watch over her, love her; and yet, after less than a moment, his arms felt numb, as if part of him knew he was essentially powerless.

"Disrespect was the message my parents constantly communicated to each other, and also how they portrayed each other to their kids. I always felt unsettled, just by virtue of the people I was living with."

Both parents worked, and Barry couldn't understand why his mother didn't take advantage of the fact that she had her own income to leave.

"I never understood the dynamic that kept them together. I felt Dad was indifferent to the kids, violent towards her. We would have done better if we had not lived with him."

He felt responsible, deep down inside where all bad feelings are kept—if he'd never existed, his parents wouldn't have had to marry, and therefore would have saved themselves and their children a whole load of grief. [Barry's in a writing group we hold every second Saturday morning at the Raging Spoon—a psychiatric-survivor-run restaurant—and he wrote a story once where he went back in time to talk his father out of this ill-fated marriage. As we listened to him read, more than a few of us sighed wistfully—if only it were possible.]

Barry started skipping school early in life, boarding the bus as usual every morning, but spending his days at the local arcade or a Chinese restaurant that served him beer. He grew even less attached to his family. Things came to a head shortly before Christmas in 1987. His father was beating his mother again in front of the children, in front of the baby sister he'd longed to protect. Barry picked up the phone and called the police, and they came and took his father away. Later, his mother got his father freed.

That was a watershed moment for him, knowing his mother would rather continue this endless battle in spite of what it was doing to her kids. Barry was arguing, pleading with her, when something snapped. He picked up a chair and flung it at the Christmas tree, decapitating it.

"I had just demonstrated to myself that I was becoming a person with destructive tendencies. I destroyed the family Christmas tree in a rage at the hypocrisy of pretence. Acting violently towards this tree—and of course it was more than just a tree—in front of my baby sister really distressed me, so I bailed."

He went to stay with a friend who'd also left a bad home, but was the smartest kid in the school he still attended. If he could do it, so could Barry. Living with his friend provided much-needed security, but Barry was learning that he could be ambushed by feelings he was trying to keep at bay; his life was getting scarier, and there seemed to be nowhere to go. He was drinking and smoking pot, not for enjoyment or pleasure, but to hold back the pain and anger that constantly threatened to consume him. Sleeping was difficult; life was difficult. He got a job dishwashing at a pizzeria from four to midnight and went to school during the day. His high school grades fluctuated between "failing to . . . above-average," depending on the subject, on his attendance, and on his ability to do the course work. Once, with no provocation, he verbally threatened a teacher he liked. He'd acted out of fear, and fear was always a trigger for him.

"I felt weird and fucked-up. I had this sense of being persecuted, that there was danger all around me."

His vice-principal suggested he go to the local hospital emergency, but Barry swore he'd see his family doctor. Though he'd trusted him in the past, Barry knew the doctor was still in touch with his family, and he didn't want to discuss what had gone on at home—how it was still affecting him. He feared the doctor would tell his parents.

When his father had wanted to belittle his mother, he'd often say she was crazy and that she needed to see a psychiatrist. For Barry, from an early age, psychiatry seemed to be a silent partner in the abuse at home. Certainly a threat.

Nonetheless, Barry kept going, finished high school, worked at minimum-wage jobs, and applied to university part-time as a mature student in philosophy. He was surprised at how easy it was and his grades were good enough that they accepted him full-time. Often, as mental health patients, we can function in the world for some time, fooling ourselves and others, faking it to make it, until the fissures widen and swallow us up.

Barry made it to his third year.

During a bio-ethics lecture, the only class that he took with one of his sisters, something the professor said was a trigger. There had been a lot of talk and press at the time about the Heritage Front, a neo-Nazi organization, setting up in Kitchener (formerly called Berlin). Sleep-deprived and delusional, Barry found it impossible to concentrate. Ideas ran like skittering mice through his head. He felt the Nazis were about to foment some evil conspiracy against society. He couldn't believe it was just his imagination; he felt compelled to speak out and to reveal the truth. Frightened but resolved, he stood up and ranted for what seemed forever, refusing to be silenced, refusing to take his seat. Finally, the teaching assistant and his sister persuaded him to leave the class, offering to drive him to hospital. He promised again to go on his own, but he just wanted to go home. He just wanted to sleep.

Barry has distrusted doctors and hospitals all his life, although he has since found one worker he trusts and likes. These days, he prefers to do his talking anonymously to what he calls Priests-in-a-Box, going into confessionals in different churches and having his say, secure that no one else will hear him but the priest, who is bound by confidentiality.

· · ·

The story of my family is one of continuing tragedy, filled with psychiatric wards and labels, suicide attempts, addictions, and too many failures to count. We were driven crazy—every curse, every blow, every corrupted touch ended up distorting us, breaking us, shaping our separate destinies.

If you didn't look too closely, and no one ever did, everything might have seemed fine, even ideal. The father went to work every day, so he must have been a good provider; the kids went off to school the way kids should, and for a long time the mother stayed home the way mothers should.

There were few visitors, no friends to speak off, just extended family dropping by once or twice a month. Sometimes, Dad would pile everyone in the car and we'd go for drives in the country, picking up bushels of apples and corn from the ubiquitous roadside stands.

The five kids were sent to Sunday School at the United Church a few blocks away to learn about right and wrong, heaven and hell, Jesus and the devil. We could relate to the ideas of damnation, hell, and punishment, though they seemed a bit watered down and sanitized in the sermons from the pulpit. Hell was where we lived, where we returned to, after the minister and the choir filed out.

Seven lives.

Four are dead now; there are only three of us left.

And we the living are uneasy, waiting for the axe to fall.

I could not love the two people who brought me home from the hospital into their family, into their war: just another tiny hostage to be used and abused for simply being.

And because I couldn't feel love for them, or from them, I felt unnatural, alien.

I was a solitary child, a loner. I lived deep down in a place where fear and pity smothered any other emotion, prevented any other attachment.

My older sister Terry and I shared a room in the house she called a concentration camp. Though I felt awful when Terry used to cry herself to sleep—deep choking sobs she'd try to muffle with her pillow as the storm of his fury raged around us—or when my mother would scream for him to stop—a terrible wrenching pity that would well up and almost stop my breathing—there was nothing I could do, and there was nowhere to run.

Sometimes my mother would scream out that he had raped her, forced her into more pregnancies, so that she couldn't ever escape. It was simple logic, then: if I hadn't been born, none of this would have happened. It was my fault, all this terror, all this pain.

I would spend a lot of time staring out the second-floor window to the street—the street that some considered picturesque, with the houses so close to us and each other—and see only studied indifference.

Once, when we still lived in Two Mountains, Terry had run crying to a neighbour's house, to beg them to make him stop beating her mom. Some crimes are bigger than others, and this telling was the biggest. Both parents beat her.

Being the wrong gender may well have been the first strike against us: four of us females, only a couple of years separating us, in the search for a son to carry on the name. The second strike was undoubtedly the cost of feeding and clothing us, these superfluous daughters. And the third seemed to be that we were never deemed worthy of the effort and sacrifice put into us.

Terry was determined to break out of the nightmare we lived in, and for her, education held the key. She studied long into the night, sticking her fingers into her ears to shut out the screams and thuds and curses that rose from downstairs. Unless, of course, it was her turn to stand before him for judgment, for a beating. (Sometimes he'd just line us all up, moving from one to the other with increasing brutality, not needing a reason, not fearing interference from neighbours or police.)

A man's home was his castle then, his children his to raise however he saw fit. He allowed his wife to take a job in the same aircraft plant he worked in, where he could watch her, control her, and be sure she wasn't planning to escape.

Terry did get out and went away to teacher's college. I had the bedroom to myself. I wrapped it around me for some illusion of safety, of apartness.

But it was my turn now to be left in charge of the others—who nicknamed me the warden—to make breakfast, to get them off to school, and to ensure chores were done.

I desperately tried to maintain appearances, the way my parents always had. It seemed to be all they cared about: how things looked.

But years of abuse had already taken root: all the curses, all the words he'd used as battering rams to destroy any sense we might have had of our worth, of our potential, had already defined us, condemned us, and set us apart.

I never considered fitting in at school an option—I would have happily settled for invisibility. I'd learned pretty quickly for a "stupid" child that any attention was potentially lethal.

School was torturous for me. I was immediately overwhelmed when I tackled things like multiplication tables, or long division, or fractions. Even in grade ten, exasperated teachers were using flashcards to try to teach me. No one said, "Of course, you're having trouble, you're scared to death of going home. You know the punishment for saying the wrong answer."

It's funny how long things stay with you. That feeling of misery and failure, that constant fear of ridicule, put on with school clothes, woven into the very fabric, part of the uniform, part of you. Teachers were more adults who saw me as a screw-up, who shook their heads or rolled their eyes or made sarcastic comments to get a laugh from the other students when in blind panic an answer would not come. There was no whisper of a hint that they might be wrong.

Some lessons we learned very well.

It's easy to teach bright, attractive, untroubled boys and girls. It's the kid that you instinctually dislike that needs you the most—the one who desperately needs reaching, needs to find something he can do that will perhaps bring the first praise ever into his life.

For me, it wasn't until the last years of my high school experience that someone, anyone, took the time to say: You have talent, you have potential. The others weren't so lucky. All they felt was condemnation, and they were determined, for a time, to live down to it.

Michael, the youngest, was breaking into cars and stealing stereos. The two girls I was supposed to "control" were doing what troubled girls have always done. I suspected these things, but telling on them was not an option, not any kind of solution.

I felt I was failing once again.

Failing them, failing my parents, failing myself.

I started to crumble, from the inside out.

Couldn't go to school, couldn't leave the house, couldn't see a way out. My nerves were stretched taut. I had prolonged fits of crying as I spent the daylight hours wandering from room to room, wringing my hands, steeped in fear.

And every evening, when his car pulled into the driveway, when Daddy brought them both back from work, I struggled to hide my disintegration from them, clenching the muscles around my mouth so forcibly that the keening sound in back of my throat would never escape.

But I had to get out, had to run, had to try.

*   *   *

Barry, Laurie, and I learned the same lessons very early: as children we were not important enough, or good enough, or bright enough, or lovable enough to cause our parents to interrupt their wars on each other and on us. The rest of the world (outsiders and extended family) would rather not know what was going on, and if they did find out, it was quite likely they would ascribe the blame to us.

We learned powerlessness; we learned that might makes right; we learned there was no safety; and with every emotional or physical blow, we learned to misshape our self-image into the one so violently drawn by our abusers. We learned that the major institutions and the people with the most impact on our lives were betraying us too.

As a group, those of us raised in this kind of environment are more attuned to detecting the Big Lie than to buying into the Big Illusion. We learned the hard way to hate the pretence and the hypocrisy, which were given more validity than truth, and that truth would be sacrificed to maintain illusions. And we learned, deep down where it counts, to hate ourselves.

In files that grow thicker with every hospital admission, the words appear often enough, couched in clinical jargon and so frequently that they have lost their power to move the helpers: abused child, hit, kicked, punched. But the words are so small and the acts so devastating, words cannot convey the weight of them.

And we who have suffered this abuse know that.

So victims stop using words. We resort to acting out the pain and despair in a mute show of need that brings only more blame and confirmation that it is indeed us who are the cause of the horrors around us. We are drowning in a deep ocean of self-loathing, within sight of the shore, within sight of people who turn away, scornful and dismissive.

The same way they always did.

When Laurie tried to speak out about what was happening to her at home and realized that no one wanted to know, she understood she was alone and lost and full of blame. No matter that somewhere in the deep recesses of her mind she recognized that the abuse she suffered was wrong, even criminal, certainly unjust. How could she sustain that knowledge when it was never confirmed by others?

Barry, perhaps already knowing what the response would be, did not speak—not until he was out of the home and out of the immediate reach of his family. He had feelings of agonized powerlessness when he held his sister in his arms. I know those feelings, too; to watch suffering is always worse than to endure it yourself.

Most of us get to a point where we stop running, stop reacting, and make some accommodation for the pain bedevilling us. For some, it may take a decade or so to experience some release; for others, it will never come, except through an overdose or after a leap in front of an onrushing subway train.

The best revenge comes from living well, or so the old expression goes. Those of us emerging from family war zones would do well to keep that in mind, rather than continuing on with the self-destruction that begins in infancy and ends when we are jailed, hospitalized, or caught up in the clutches of addictions.

The tyranny of the majority view of "family" silences, cripples, and condemns. As early as grade school, children should be given the tools and the right to speak up. The curriculum should support studies of different kinds of families, and explain what a child can do when his parents are violent and hurtful. It should help students get a sense of how abused children feel guilty and bad, and how those feelings are likely to play out, if we're not watchful. School officials and extended families must not turn a blind eye to clear evidence of abuse, believing all parents to be wonderful, loving creatures who are occasionally burdened with the "bad seed" child.

Mental health professionals must learn the silent language of behaviour, rather than reject those who are troublesome and non-communicative. Counsellors can channel a victim's anger to fuel a drive for success in life, for revenge of the best sort. Children emerging from violence desperately crave warmth and acceptance and understanding. They take to it like fish to water. The problem is, even in the caring professions, they so rarely encounter it. Psychiatry is too concerned with the search for the biological and physiological causes of mental illness to address these basic emotional needs, and so it fails us. We are more than chemical disorders—we are individuals smothered with pain, and we need a human response to suffering if we are to overcome it.

2.

Bred
in the
Bone

In this society, it doesn't pay to be too different, though how you can be anything other than who you are escapes me.
—a Parkdale survivor

Practitioners of psychiatry often speak in strong, confident voices, secure in their knowledge of pathology and their ability to re-trace its history. They rarely look, however, at the profession's past mistakes and missteps. Such a collective denial does not recognize the harm that was done "back then" in the name of mental health. Instead, the focus is on the present and on the very promising, very lucrative future. There are always exceptions, thank God, but the status and income of psychiatrists work against self-examination and self-doubt.

Mental health patients learn at an early age to trust professional experts, especially those with "doctor" in front of their names. The families who bring patients to psychiatrists find great relief in the evident expertise, in the framed diplomas, in the beards and pipes, and in the professionalism. They want a label assigned to the odd behaviour they've witnessed in their family members. They are sure the doctors must know, and they must know what's best.

Survivors, on the other hand, have a jaundiced view of medical models, past and present. They have a strong sense of continuity and identity with the patients who have gone before. They understand what these men and women have endured in search of a cure. They understand that they have frightened themselves and others by responding aloud to the voices in their heads and that they have been convicted and incarcerated with no hope of release, simply for being diagnosed as mentally ill.

Thanks to the efforts of researchers, for example, we now know that many of the women who were shut away as mentally ill in provincial institutions in the fifties, sixties, and seventies had been victims of sexual abuse. Their complaints weren't heard or they weren't believed. And we can only wonder how women who wanted something other from life, who perhaps weren't cut out to be mothers, wives, and caregivers, felt when they were told that their negative feelings were evidence of mental disease. They, too, were locked up in their best interests, while their families backed away. Research also shows that not so very long ago, women who were stuck in abusive situations, such as my mother's, and who went to professionals for help were given scripts for Valium so they could endure their tortured lives in stoic silence.

This chapter looks at children who were raised by a parent who was labelled as chronically mentally ill. *Chronic* is a word that is being challenged by survivors these days, since it defines the care they received more than the label they carry. *Serious mental illness* is the term that now refers to schizophrenia, manic depression, depression, or any illness that has a profound and lengthy negative impact on the individual experiencing it.

There was a time when psychiatry blamed the mothers if their sons or daughters became psychotic. They traced it back to coldness, or double messages, or withholding of affection, and added a huge burden of guilt to the grief these women already bore. Now psychiatrists see behaviour as a result of biological and physiological factors. The notion of inheriting a psychiatric disease does seem to make some sense, though—the survivors in this chapter are now coping themselves with diagnoses of serious mental illness. But we are complex, messy, confusing creations that defy easy categorization. Our needs are equally complex and psychiatrists must not fall into the trap of only seeing what their education tells them is there.

On the other hand, who's to say what is predetermined and what is learned behaviour? If you were raised by an abusive parent, you'll have difficulty with relationships and trust throughout your life. If you were raised by an alcoholic parent, chances are you'll copy that way of coping with life. If you were raised in a chaotic household, where a parent was often taken away, you will not feel safe and secure.

·   ·   ·

I met the Grays while I was working in the Parkdale drop-in, Parc (Parkdale Activity and Recreation Centre)—a place for "mental patients" to wile away their days. Alan and Beverly took better physical care with their appearance than those who were too impoverished and desperate to be able to pull themselves together. Clean clothes, hair always washed—if you didn't look too closely you might wonder if they were in the wrong place. Though Alan took his antipsychotic medication religiously, he still lived with delusions and still talked to the voices in his head. When he came in without Beverly, it was a bit disconcerting to see him conversing with no one we could see. The other members were a little spooked and avoided him, so staff would make a point to get him into a card game, to get him to talk about everyday things. He appreciated this—though he was unable to express it—and his symptoms would diminish for the time we were with him.

Beverly must have been beautiful in her youth. She was still quite striking, though now she defined sadness. Her whole body, even her facial features seemed weighed down, pulled by powerful forces from her past. She could smile and even laugh, but these brief flashes faded too quickly.

They'd had a child together, Cheryl. Sometimes they'd bring her to the drop-in, and their pride and delight in her was obvious. Cheryl was quiet and as watchful as her mom, and she could get lost in the wake of the others if we didn't make a special effort to include her.

The request the couple made to my co-worker Paul Quinn and me to be witnesses at their wedding came out of the blue. They'd never asked for anything before. Many of the people at Parc had no one outside the mental patient community left in their lives. Too much time had been spent "away," locked up in hospitals and absent from families with more problems than resources to deal with them. If I'd thought about it at all, I assumed Alan and Beverly were already married. However, they wanted their child to have legitimacy and were going to City Hall to make the relationship official. They were both beaming that day. Beverly looked radiant in a smart dress and Alan had on a suit. Even Paul had dug up a sports jacket to wear. After the words were spoken and the papers signed, we had a glass of wine to celebrate. Cheryl watched everything closely from her seat on Daddy's lap.

Seventeen years later, Cheryl called. She'd found my name and Paul's on her parents' marriage certificate. Her hesitant voice asked if I remembered her and brought back memories of the little waif with long blonde hair, large eyes, and a perpetually runny nose, sticking close to her mother in the chaos of the Parc drop-in. I had wondered through the years what her life was like, what she thought about, if she'd made it through her childhood relatively intact. She was calling, she said, because she knew I was a survivor activist and she was looking for information about mental illness, the kind of information you don't get from psychiatrists. At twenty-one, she was carrying enough guilt, anger, and confusion to last several lifetimes. She also had a lot of insight into the lives of chronic mental patients, her parents' world.

Cheryl remembered Parc as a very inviting place. Her parents, who didn't know many people, seemed to have friends there because "everybody knew everybody." Her own house, however, was often very empty and very quiet.

"My parents would just sit, and stare ahead, and smoke. Sometimes my dad would watch television. I was a noisy kid, at least when I was home. I liked to sing and dance, and make my mom laugh. I'd put on shows, making up characters and using different voices, even assigning them roles. My dad would sometimes dance with me. He loved dancing, and we'd manage by him putting my feet on his."

Alan and Beverly both got up every morning to get Cheryl's breakfast and see her off to school.

"The only other role they had in their lives, besides being mental patients, was to be my parents."

And they were good parents. She knew she was loved with a very unselfish love—not that either of them was demonstrative, but it was how they spoke to her, what they did for her. They were poor, of course, but even if there was no toilet paper in the house at times, there was always food. At Christmas there were presents for her even though there was no money to buy for each other. They lived in poor areas, moving frequently when her father's paranoia about the neighbours grew too much for him (Cheryl went to ten different elementary schools), but compared to the kids she hung out with, she had model parents.

"They didn't drink, didn't beat me, and didn't do drugs. They taught me the blacks and whites, right from wrong, good from bad, and I filled in the greys. I had manners. I was always well dressed in clean clothes. I was well fed. I was never left alone. I always felt safe. I socialized myself, probably through television, so I had friends."

There was always a small surprise waiting for her when she got back from school, a chocolate bar or something special. When Cheryl brought her friends home and the kids would put on music and dance, her mom would get a sparkle in her eyes: "I think she was very proud of me."

Cheryl knew they both took medication and that they were different. But they masked their bad feelings—she only saw her mother cry twice. It was harder for her father, who would respond to the voices in his head or to what he thought the television might be telling him. He never had a bad psychotic episode that she witnessed. If he felt himself slipping, he'd go to the hospital.

She knew people in the neighbourhood thought her folks were weird, especially since they would see her off to school from the balcony and then stay there for the rest of the day drinking tea. Some thought there was something else in those mugs, but there wasn't. Cheryl says it was the lifestyle, the role, of the mental patient at the time: take your pills in the morning, sit around and

wait to take them at lunch, and then wait some more for the
supper and bedtime pills.

There were moments, though, when Cheryl would see clearly
that her parents were in pain. One year she was given a Polaroid
camera, and she took her mom's picture when she wasn't aware
she was being photographed.

"It struck me, looking at it, how sad and far away she looked."

As she got older, Cheryl became more aware of the penalties
of being different and that she had no magic to heal her parents.
She also got a sense of what should be and of what was missing.

They had just moved again, Alan being certain of the gathering hostility of his immediate neighbours. Perhaps he was
picking up on negative vibrations from those who were frightened at the idea of living next door to people who suffered
from mental illness. As buttons and T-shirts declare, even
paranoids have real enemies. However, this meant Cheryl had
to start over at yet another school. The kids there were different from the friends she used to make; they listened to different
music and wore different clothes. In her last neighbourhood,
there were a lot of black children: hip-hop was big and so was
"ghetto" clothing. The new place was, or seemed to be, solidly
middle class and white. Cheryl started skipping school, and
her parents understood fear and difference too well to force her
to go.

"If I'd tell my mom I didn't want to go to gym class, that it
was scary for me, she'd say, it would be scary for her too. Then
I'd get mad and yell at her that she should be telling me to go!"

It was a confusing and rebellious time for Cheryl, but she couldn't say what was wrong. She would argue with her dad, challenging his beliefs that everything he saw or heard on television was true. She describes herself as having been a bit of a know-it-all. The school principal called her house. Workers were sent to talk to the family, and her parents—and Cheryl—hated it. They found it threatening and intrusive.

"I refused to talk to the people they sent, hoping they'd go away. Sometimes I'd pretend to be sleeping. More workers came. It didn't take them long to realize my parents were different, and I knew they were judging them. My parents couldn't express themselves the way they wanted to, especially my dad, suffering with schizophrenia. My mom was very sensitive. She had a lot of issues, bitterness, and anger; things would come out when she was depressed or that made her seem more depressed than she was. The workers got the impression that I was taking care of my parents, rather than the other way around. I learned to just agree with them, or I'd just pretend to sleep through their 'visits,' hoping they would stop asking questions and go away."

A worker told her there was a place that could help her get back to school, that she could choose to stay or go once she saw it, and that she would like it there. She remembers thinking, when she arrived in tow, "Holy shit, this is a psychiatric ward!" There was no choice, of course. Even though she was not clinically depressed and not a danger to herself or others, she was quickly admitted. She was put through a battery of diagnostic tests and learned that there was a significant chance that she might develop an illness like her parents. Watching the other children play out their problems in self-destructive ways, she started having panic attacks, and began to wonder about herself. The hospital kept her a month, and then returned her to her family, but a lot of damage had been done.

After meeting with her social worker, principal, and parents, her teacher explained to the students in Cheryl's class that they had to be nice to her because she had "emotional problems."

"That totally fucked up any chance I had of making friends in school."

She continued to skip school.

And the system continued to intervene.

Decisions and arrangements were made, and at twelve she was sent to a foster home outside the city—a terrible move that left her with a huge burden of guilt for the destruction of her little family. In retrospect, Cheryl believes that her initial truancy was learned behaviour: if she had a problem, she would run from it, the way her dad did with his frequent moving. If only the workers had given her and her parents the tools they needed, they may have been able to stay together.

There was no comfort in the assessment home that was her first placement. The foster kids Cheryl lived with were emotionally scarred and wrecked, with parents who had deliberately hurt and destroyed them. She felt like an outsider. At some point, she decided that if she was going to be crazy, she might as well act the part. She shaved her head, started drinking, and even tried smoking pot. But she couldn't hold her booze and weed "made her twitch." She didn't like feeling out of control.

She continued to avoid school—the only way she could protest what had happened to her—until she found herself (in her third placement) in a more supportive environment with a family she liked.

*   *   *

Cheryl's mother, Beverly, had also been a ward of Children's Aid. In spite of this, for a time she had worked as a secretary at the University of Toronto, and she had married a young man from Malta with whom she had a son. The family history is a bit murky here—either her husband's return to Malta with their child precipitated her first psychotic episode or her illness resulted in him leaving. Undoubtedly, losing Cheryl sparked memories of grief and failure in Beverly, feelings that were aggravated when her now-grown son tracked her down. His life had been difficult; he'd also been placed in a state institution in England when his father had a child by a new wife.

Cheryl, however, was excited to learn that she had a half-brother—a big brother, who came to visit her at her foster home. She wasn't aware that her mother was drowning; she felt Cheryl and her brother now had each other, and that they could look after each other. Beverly was plagued with regret and self-blame for the pain she had caused them and she died

of an overdose when Cheryl was eighteen. Alan quickly went
downhill with no one to look after him and he was placed in
a "home."

Cheryl began to suffer from depression. At this time, she had
"graduated" to a kind of halfway house with other young women
who were making the transition from CAS to independence.
Workers were still watching for signs of mental illness, and this
undermined Cheryl's efforts to stand alone. She decided that if
she stayed any longer with CAS, she'd end up like her peers
who were begging or hooking on downtown streets, living in
temporary shelters, and taking drugs. It was a scary decision, but
she admitted herself to a psychiatric hospital, fearing that the
depression was engulfing her.

Cheryl was very lucky. She encountered nurses and psychiatrists who reassured her, recognized her intelligence, and encouraged her to learn about psychiatric diagnosis and medications.
They even sent her to groups to help her become more assertive.
She met patients who were working professionals and whose
illnesses were considered interruptions in their lives rather than
lifelong limitations. She remembers being very ready to leave
when the staff set a discharge date, and she recalls a patient saying
to her, "You must be leaving soon. You're smiling a lot, and this
isn't a place for people who smile."

Cheryl had a new determination and she made it clear: "I
refuse to have a shitty life; I refuse to be in and out of supportive
housing; I refuse to be a mental patient; I refuse to become an
alcoholic or a drug addict. I am going to break the cycle."

Cheryl's determination to break the cycle saved her. Most of the people I'd known at Parc when I worked there, however, had so little fight left in them.

·   ·   ·

There were so damn many of us (though I was supposed to be different now—I was staff). They crowded the place, filling it with smoke and deep guttural coughing; they were hungry and they were dirty and they were broken. They were called members here, not mental patients, though that identity was inescapable, constantly betrayed by their poverty, their peculiar, stiff-legged gait, and the emptiness in their eyes.

Most lived in boarding and rooming houses in the neighbourhood, places much like the one I'd just left, and they were the lucky ones. Others lived on the street, or under bridges, or spent nights wandering from hostel to hostel in search of a place to lay their heads. All came together in a neighbourhood that resented their presence and often feared them. Their dilapidated residences affected property values; negative publicity branded the area a psychiatric ghetto.

Surrounded, drowning in the immediate need for food, clothing, and housing for those recently evicted—lost drug cards, stolen medication—the seven years I worked there rushed by in a flurry of doing for. But they kept coming—new people all the time, new problems, new street drugs, new street diseases.

It was insane.

People who had been locked up on the back wards of provincial hospitals for their own protection, who had been labelled chronically mentally ill, were simply thrown to the dogs. For-profit landlords, dealers, everyone was eager to take the pittance that made up their income, their government pension.

And people got mad at them. Harassed them, beat them up, drove them out of stores and restaurants.

They should be sent back to hospital, said the more refined: they'll be taken care of there; they'll be safe.

And we wouldn't have to see them anymore.

•　•　•

When I first met Allan Strong, he was an advocate for families of the mentally ill and he worked for the provincial Depression and Manic Depression organization. Allan is sturdily built and good-looking. Articulate, intense, and funny, he spoke passionately of the need for survivors and families to work together to make the system a better place. He understood the bewilderment and guilt children feel when they watch, but don't understand, the disintegration of a mentally ill parent.

Allan's father came from "a small WASP town in Eastern Ontario, where he was raised to do the right thing." He describes his parents as oil and water—two people who, like Barry's parents, should never have married. His dad was a travelling salesman and his job selling first life insurance, then detergent for

Proctor and Gamble, and then vitamins for a pharmaceutical company kept him on the road a lot during the week.

"It seemed like my mother saved up all the frustration she felt during the week while he was gone, and then she'd come in Friday night all liquored up and ready to fight. My father was an abused spouse, emotionally, verbally, even physically, those times she'd throw things at him."

Allan's mother was often still in bed when the kids came home from school so he and his sister, the oldest kids, prepared meals, made beds, and cleaned the house. Allan never brought friends home, preferring their places to his. In high school, he stayed late for student council or drama club or even sports, anything rather than go home.

None of this saved him from reacting to his home life. He was fourteen when he started drinking, smoking, and occasionally shoplifting. His mother had introduced him to booze when he was ten or eleven: she would sit him down, pour him some sherry, and make him her drinking buddy, dumping her problems and disappointments on his young shoulders. Much later, he learned she'd been seeing a psychiatrist since she was twenty, although she was thirty-six when she really "went off the deep end." He only spoke once of his trials at home. Late in high school he did try to tell his girlfriend about his mother's illness. Her response was, "You won't catch it too, will you?"

His mother also had a bit of a religious mania.

"She'd believe she was Jesus Christ. I remember getting a sense of wrongness when she'd make us sit around the kitchen table and read the Bible by candlelight. To me, religion was something that happened at church, not like this."

Sometimes when Allan came home, his mother would be lying in the street and an ambulance would take her away. His father had a sense of responsibility that kept him hanging in, but it was his mother who initiated the final separation. She moved into an apartment and took his sisters with her. They didn't stay long—relationships with their mother were too difficult. When Allan was getting ready to go to college, his mom—now lonely—asked him to stay with her.

"Actually, what she said was, if you stay with me, I'll always make sure there's beer in the fridge."

He had to move to Toronto to make the break, but even that wasn't far enough away. He was frequently called home to deal with his mother's crises. He had learned to handle his memories and moods by drinking, until he "could down a twenty-sixer of whisky and go looking for more." If he felt himself slipping into depression, he'd withdraw, drink, and be melancholic for a few weeks.

"It was how I numbed my pain. It was convenient, even sanctioned, once I was of age."

By now he was married with two children and his wife delivered an ultimatum: stop drinking or risk losing his family. He stopped, but his "coping mechanism was gone." His first episode developed gradually over four months, so that even he was not aware that he was slipping away. He wasn't going to work and had stopped phoning to tell them he wasn't coming in. He'd be up all night pacing, getting really paranoid, hearing voices. He wouldn't, couldn't, talk to his wife or children.

He discovered cutting.

"It really felt like such a release, the physical pain lets you know you're alive, still alive. I was watching myself do the cut— I felt like it wasn't me. But it also served as an alarm for me, like 'Hey buddy, what the hell are you doing?'"

Six months after the death of his mother, Allan was in hospital and eventually labelled with manic depression. He feels it's significant that he was about the same age as she had been when she had her first big break with reality; he was thirty-five.

Allan is ambivalent about his mother. Sometimes he speaks with a poignant mix of pride and confusion about the friends she made in later life and how they loved her. But the anger is there too, just below the surface, for the woman who left him a legacy of pain.

He had three hospitalizations in two years. Cutting preceded all of them.

"I was even having delusions that were similar to my mom's. You know, there's a religious revival happening on the planet, and I have to cut myself to release the toxins from my body, to purify myself."

Allan doesn't want his children to be afraid the way he was watching his mother spiral out of control. He doesn't want to put them through that, and when they're old enough, he intends to talk to them about his diagnosis and treatment. He's created a network of support for himself and is part of the Mennonite community in Kitchener-Waterloo through his marriage, where he has found people who are there for him.

Unlike the professionals, I'm not sure that he simply inherited a disease from his mother. So many other factors are at play here—guilt, anger, and fear—that to reduce it to genetics is probably an oversimplification. What matters most is that Allan has love, joy, and friendship in his life now and he doesn't want to lose that, so he is taking all the right steps to keep himself going. His medications help, and he is reaching out to help others.

•　•　•

I met Jill Stainsby in downtown Vancouver in the mid-nineties, while I was doing some work for the Greater Vancouver Mental Health Services agency. An imposing woman who radiated calm and quiet competence, Jill identified herself as a psychiatric survivor, but I didn't ask about her background at that time. I suppose if I'd thought about it, I would have assumed depression or even bipolar disorder, so I was quite surprised when I later learned that she had the mother of all heavy-duty labels: paranoid schizophrenia.

"It runs in the family," she said, matter-of-factly.

Jill's parents were solidly middle class; her dad was a journalist and her birth mother was a librarian.

"I had one father and three mothers, serially, and I'm the eldest of seven children."

Her parents wanted the best for their kids in terms of good schools and opportunities, and raised them in Vancouver's West End. Jill was five years old when her mother had her first psychotic break. She remembers being told by the nanny that the children (her mother had had three kids in four years) were all going to collect cherries from the tree that stood on a small hill in their front yard. Jill glanced back in time to see her mother being escorted out of the house by two men; she was resisting, trying to turn back, her arms flailing as she struggled.

"Riverview Psychiatric Hospital actually had a van back then that would come and collect people."

It's unusual for middle-class patients to have their first hospitalization at a provincial institution; generally that's reserved for the poor and chronically ill. But, as a student, Jill's aunt had toured the Crease Building at Riverview, a state-of-the-art facility, and she had thought it was a wonderful place.

"My aunt is very clear now that she was not right about that."

It was the start of a series of confinements.

"Once, when I was quite young, we went out on a 'Sunday drive.' I did not realize that my mother was delusional, though the adults must have, because the drive led us directly to Riverview and Mom was left there. It was incredibly surprising and stressful to me. I froze in fear."

Her mother wouldn't be held for long, since she "had a survivor skill I don't possess: even when unmedicated she could revert to sanity." That meant she'd be released, and the extended family would deliver the children back to her. Jill thinks someone may have tried to explain her mother's illness, since she "was the only kid in grade three who could spell schizophrenia," but she can't recollect who, when, or even what was said.

She does recall the time she first blew the whistle on her mom. She was on her way to church camp. She was eleven and had already learned to watch for the signs of what others called psychosis—when her mother would talk to the air or become lost in delusions. Worried about the children she'd left behind, she made a phone call to relatives, a "mom's crazy again" call. She was angry, because every time her mom "went off," she and her brothers and sisters would lose their mother's support and whatever stability they'd managed to achieve since the last episode.

Jill attended eight different elementary schools, which made friendships impossible, although she was a strong student. School was a much more stable environment than home. Home was always in chaos, and Jill had to become a caretaker with no time to deal with her own needs, her own murky feelings of anger and frustration.

"I think I was a bitter, sarcastic child."

After her graduation from grade twelve, she says, "Home left me." Her father and his third wife took off for Europe, and Jill was on her own. In university, she completed nine credits towards an anthropology degree, and then left to work in a series of manual labour jobs. She worked on fishing boats and managed the graders on the "slime line" at a Vancouver fish plant, washing the gutted catch. In her spare time, she tore into life with great gusto—"sex, drugs, and rock 'n' roll"—and British Columbia in

the late sixties and early seventies was the place to do it. By the
time she was in her early twenties, she was hanging out with a
large group of friends and living in a truck parked at a marina.

It wouldn't be long until she crashed and burned.

Her first mental health crisis occurred in the context of
coming out as a lesbian.

"Many of us were locked up then, since gay or lesbian identi-
ties were diagnosed as illnesses by the American Psychiatric
Association until 1975. Mental health services can be incredibly
ham-handed, directive, and judgmental, as well as sexist and
homophobic, and this can be hugely hurtful and damaging.
Dishonesty may have been a smarter move at the time."

Her "self-esteem was in the gutter" and she was struggling
to come out about her sexuality. She did not connect her
experience to a genetic factor. She knew she was unhappy and
angry about her chaotic upbringing, that she'd had a lot of
pain, and that she'd partied too much, but she had "a wilful
blindness that served me well. The synaptic link failed with
me." Though her first hospitalization was in 1976, she didn't
become aware of her label of paranoid schizophrenia until
1987, after she'd racked up enough positives in life, including
her two university degrees, not to feel that it was a death
sentence.

"I went, oh, of course, oh shit."

She remembers being shocked that the mental health professionals on the wards she stayed on had no clue about what was
going on with her.

"They don't understand the concept of being all broken inside, what Anaïs Nin used to call the 'shattered mirror' within."

Jill was determined to handle her diagnosis in a different way than her mother had.

"She had only one string in her bow, the 'system is hurting me, the system is hurting me.'"

Jill educated herself; she took her medications religiously (even to the point of giving herself the IMAP intermuscular injections before that drug was discontinued by its maker for being unprofitable); and she kept watch on herself. And she keeps living, growing, working, and studying.

I was in Vancouver recently for a conference on women and mental health and saw a remarkable video titled *Within These Walls* that Jill produced on inpatients, including her mother, at Riverview and other psychiatric hospitals. I was reminded of how far we've come, which is so difficult to see when so much remains to be done. Jill's mom wears the effects of years of antipsychotics on her face, but she remains a strong, articulate woman, bemused by the changes she's seen. In 1994, Jill got a part-time job at Riverview, a hospital she'd managed to avoid becoming a patient in, working with a psychiatric nurse to coordinate patient relations. Being a psychiatric survivor counted as much in getting the job as her university education, and during her time there she helped to implement the new *Charter of Patient Rights*.

Jill remembers telling her mother a story about the then head of the hospital, whom she referred to as Dianne [Macfarlane]. Her mother's mouth dropped open in surprise that her daughter, a sometime "mental patient," could call the president of the hospital by her first name and not be threatened with four-point restraints.

"The staff were more institutionalized than the patients, and much of my time was spent proving and proving and proving to them that they weren't doing anything differently than the way they'd done things for years, though they often felt they were [much more progressive]," says Jill. In six years, she and her partner processed 1,500 complaints, mainly to do with being treated—or not treated—with dignity and respect, access to the grounds, requests for change of worker and medication reviews, and abuse of power.

These days, Jill works at the Vancouver Coastal Authority, coordinating a peer-support worker-training program and other consumer initiatives, and she is pursuing a master's degree in social work at the University of British Columbia. She has a full life with many friends, likes to square dance, has two cats, and a nice, orderly apartment. Above all, she is achieving for herself and for her community.

Jill will feel a tremendous sense of accomplishment when she finishes her degree; if she had given up, given in to this illness, the failure would haunt her for the rest of her life. The education of psychiatric survivors in the social services, nursing, research, and psychology fields will improve the mental health system, as people with direct knowledge and experience of their institutions, such as Jill, take up positions.

Many survivors are returning to school, just as those with physical disabilities are making strides and conquering obstacles in the physical realm. For some, education reshapes self-image in positive ways, as they learn they are more capable and brighter than they were led to believe. Medications can make reading and retention difficult; there may be a need for more time to complete assignments or the right to carry less of a course load; students may need to take time off once in a while for self-care. None of this should come with a penalty. There are many hurdles, but great rewards.

Jill has thought a lot about what her mother and all the men and women in her video endured. Imagine their fear, locked away for months, for years. Imagine their rage at the violation of their bodies, their minds. Imagine their devastating powerlessness. So some of them drank, choosing a gentler poison than the pills they were given, to mute the resentment, anger, and defeat. There was no room left in them for their families—there was only pain.

"This was her reality: she was first hospitalized at twenty-seven (I was five at the time), in 1958. The therapies she and others endured included long-term, forced confinement, Thorazine, Stelazine, and chlorpromazine—the original creators of the 'psychiatric shuffle,' and of many patients' unconscious ability to stare vacantly ahead for hours, and/or drool. They also included insulin comas and electroconvulsive shock therapy. My mom resisted them and other treatments and medications all her adult life. She was significantly damaged, both by illness (psychosis) and addictions, as well as treatment."

It was the families, innocently trusting to the experts in mental illness, who kept sending these men and women back. It was the experts who kept them confined. Institutionalization kept them childlike, self-absorbed, dependent, acting out. That ensured that all they would ever be were mental patients, and that their children would run into problems later on, genetics or not. There were no rights, no survivor movements, certainly no role models, or questioning of what was being done to them in the name of mental health.

Go into any provincial mental hospital today, and you can still meet those who bear the burden of the medical model of psychiatric practice. Their bodies jerk with the long-term side effects of antipsychotic medications. They stopped growing as people long ago, defeated by the "care" given them. Their only friends are paid staff, and their only pleasures a bummed cigarette or cup of coffee.

Survivors raising children now, however, can avoid recycling their illness. We have more control over our lives and more awareness of the responsibilities once removed from us. We have more say in our treatment and can hold on to jobs. We can give our children the childhoods we wished for, and take pride in what they accomplish. We can talk with them, reassure them, love them, caution them, and discipline them so that they can grow straight and tall. They should never need to walk into the emergency ward of the local hospital for help with their minds.

3.

Blindsided

*The life of every man is a diary in which he means to write one
story, and writes another; and his humblest hour is when he
compares the volume as it is with what he vowed to make it.*
—Sir J.M. Barrie

Sometimes the life that is comfortably laid out, that looks promising and exciting, is derailed—derailed so badly we think we can
never get back to it. We find we don't fit in; we are not like everyone else. Sometimes our behaviour grows increasingly bizarre, at
home, at school. Teachers judge us and judge us harshly, and we
internalize every negative word, every exasperated look. We are
too young to understand that life holds no guarantees and that
there is no intrinsic fairness. We become angry or frightened, or
both, and look for a way to calm the turmoil inside. It can be
with prescribed or illicit drugs or through a bottle—whatever
way, it's something we reach for that's out there, not within us.

The people in this chapter were blindsided by circumstance. Here are their stories.

•   •   •

For Dan Carter and Julie Flatt, home life was wonderful and accepting. They had both had parents who loved and supported them—solid starts, one would think. I met Dan, a tall, slender, aristocratic-looking man, while being interviewed about books I had written, *The War at Home* and *Bound by Duty*. Dan hosts a television show on CHEX-TV, and he works really hard to get it right. He actually reads the books he reviews, for one thing. His professionalism shows in every detail, from the look of the set to the questions he asks. It is unusual for writers to be moved by the person showcasing them, but after Dan gave me a glimpse into his life during a commercial break, I was impatient to finish the interview and learn more about this man.

Dan lucked out really early, although it didn't look like good fortune at the time. His mother died from a brain aneurysm shortly after giving birth to him, and his father, a soldier in the Canadian military, was unable to care for him. So the first foster home Dan was sent to by Children's Aid became his real home. Charlie and Isabel Carter had fostered about fourteen babies, and they had three children of their own—two boys and a girl. On February 14, 1962, at the age of two, Dan was officially adopted into their family, with the blessing of his new brothers and sister. Michael, the eldest, was almost nineteen years older than Dan; his sister was twelve, and the youngest, David, was eight years old. They lived in Agincourt, east of Toronto, though it was a very different place then than now.

"It was a wonderful place to grow up. There were only about twelve houses in a ten-mile radius, and we had a horse farm across the street from us."

Dan's problems started when he was sent to kindergarten, and they continued for the rest of his school years.

"Very early, people were scratching their heads over me, saying this kid just isn't getting it. He doesn't know right from left, up from down. By the time I hit grade one, they were sending me for all these physical tests, checking on my vision and hearing. I couldn't spell, couldn't read. Either there was something wrong with me or I was just lazy."

People didn't know about dyslexia back then. Schools tended to divide kids into those who learned and those who didn't. Dan spent a lot of time with his desk out in the hallway, not because of disruptive behaviour, but because his teachers were exasperated with him. [I frequently ask members of groups I work with, marginalized men and women, how they learn best. Not surprisingly, everyone talks about one-on-one teaching with someone warm and gentle who doesn't become impatient or mean when something is not understood the first or second time.] Dan was frustrated too and beginning to feel very isolated. He was kept back in grade one and felt even lonelier.

"I wanted normality. I wanted to be like everyone else."

He went home for lunch every day crying, and his mother was always there to encourage and support him.

"She'd tell me I was okay, that everything was all right. Although she didn't understand what was wrong either, she was on my side."

His mother battled the teachers' attitudes, declaring that her son was very bright, but they couldn't see that. Over the years, Dan got more and more angry with his teachers and with the system. He knew he was smart because "my mother told me" and because "as long as things were presented to me orally, I could get them. I could argue and debate well, yet they could still make me feel stupid that I couldn't learn the way they wanted." For Dan, even the solace of his home could not protect him from the corrosive effects of failing at school.

He was twelve when he started drinking. He uses dates as touchstones: the day he was adopted; the day he took his first drink in July 1972. That month, his brother Michael, who was an undercover cop, died in a mysterious motorcycle accident near the family cottage. The family was devastated, and Dan was left with a "whole slew of things to deal with." There was the continuing agony of school and worse, there was a big secret he'd told no one about. At the age of seven, he'd been raped by a male stranger at the local gas station.

He was also just coming under the influence of a group of boys who were already familiar with the joys of alcohol and who were quite willing to share. Not only did booze help him to escape the life he was leading, but it also made him really witty and funny—he'd found a way to get the acceptance and appreciation he craved.

"I was programmed for the next eighteen years. That's how it works with booze. First it introduces you to its joys, and then it slowly, slowly draws you in. As your body makes chemical changes to adjust to what you're pouring into it, you need more and more, and then you're no longer self-medicating, you're just co-existing with alcohol."

He worked at different jobs over the years, moving from one to another because of the drinking. He tried acting for a long time, and then sold clothing and shoes. As well, there was all the financial havoc that comes with drinking way too much—non-payment of rent, using one credit card to pay off another, missing car payments. Pretty much everyone he knew had told him at one time or another that he was an alcoholic. His response was to say, "Fuck off, you haven't lived my life." His family was very frustrated with him and grew distant.

All the more reason to drink.

Sexually assaulted at seven, afraid to tell, afraid it meant he was gay, abused at school—for Dan, every day was misery. Did this adopted child feel he was letting down the family he lived with? He had had every advantage in his life and his siblings were successful—he should have been achieving, not screwing up. What on earth was wrong with him?

Addiction is now seen as an illness, not a character weakness. Someone who drinks himself or herself to death is hardly a paragon of mental stability. Not so long ago, however, the fields of mental health and addiction were carefully separated, and labels could be used to avoid admitting people to the programs they sought out. If a psychiatrist felt the individual's main problem was addiction, he or she could be sent away. Likewise, mental illness could bar people from accessing what they needed. Detoxes often refused to allow clients to continue taking psychiatric medications while they were confined for alcohol or drug abuse. In Ontario, mental health and addiction have been brought under one umbrella—a late but necessary development in care.

Like so many of us made uncomfortable in our own skins, Dan turned to alcohol to remove the blame, the guilt, and the sense of difference he felt. It smoothed out the rough edges, brought him friends, and gave him a degree of acceptance. How could it be bad? Dan's struggle with substance abuse ran its course for eighteen destructive years. How he finally took control of his life is discussed in Chapter 7. Perhaps Dan would have benefited from early counselling, but, as Julie Flatt learned, this may not have helped.

•   •   •

Julie Flatt has the driest sense of humour of anyone I've met. It has been a life-saving quality. Julie and I have known each other for a long time. We've worked together on projects and listened to each other's speeches. Julie stands tall, both literally and in the survivor movement. Since 1991 she has been the provincial development consultant and peer advocacy liaison for the Consumer/Survivor Development Initiative, an organization funded by the Ontario Ministry of Health, and she is now acting director of the Ontario Peer Development Initiative.

Raised in Newmarket, Ontario, Julie was the fourth of eight children, three of whom died within days of their birth. Her mother suffered from rheumatoid arthritis and had to be hospitalized often. Her father had to quit work and stay home to take care of the children. Julie felt a constant threat that her mother wouldn't be returning.

When she was four, Julie began to choke on her food and to wash her hands repeatedly. Then, when she started going school, she ran back and forth up the street to her house to kiss her mom goodbye over and over again, perhaps ten or twenty times, before she felt able to leave her neighbourhood. By the time she was eight, she had developed a fear of swallowing her tongue and wouldn't swallow her saliva, but she didn't tell anyone. She began to have acute anxiety attacks. At fourteen, she had a terrible feeling that she had taken someone's life—she didn't know whose or how.

Her mother wondered if 999 (the old address of the Queen Street Mental Health Centre) might help, but Julie pleaded with her not to take her there. Everyone referred to that place as the nuthouse. Julie had a real fear of being sent there, especially since her brother-in-law's mother had died in Whitby Psychiatric Hospital, the label of schizophrenia going with her to the grave. Julie did agree to see someone at a hospital, however, and she was put on Stelazine and Halcion: "Halcion had me up all night singing Beatles tunes, and I don't even like the Beatles."

Julie could not continue on the drugs. Later, she and her mom met with a psychiatrist at another hospital. After a while, he asked Julie to leave the room so he could speak privately with her mother. Julie refused, and her anger still comes through: "I refused. After all, it's my frigging life! I can still hear him saying to me, 'You're a spoiled little bitch.'"

As mental health patients, our first experience of professional help can determine our response for the rest of our psychiatric careers. When we go for help, we're at our most vulnerable and the last thing we need is someone looking down his nose at us and passing blind judgment. I remember hearing with open-mouthed disbelief my own psychiatrist telling me I was spoiled, while images of beatings danced uncondemned in my head. How can you believe anything they tell you after that? Shrinks are the flagships of the mental health system: when they blow their credibility with their patients out of the water, what's left?

Shock treatment was recommended for Julie. [It must have been the treatment of choice for spoiled females, since it was also suggested for me.]

She declined.

"I am very blessed that my parents were very cautious. They listened to my wishes. They gave a damn. My mom knew something bad was wrong with me, but my parents knew I knew what made me feel better."

Julie knows too many survivors whose parents didn't listen, parents who grew angry and frustrated when their children refused treatment that would make them better and keep them safe. These parents couldn't recognize that the price their children would pay for "stability" was too high, too emotionally and spiritually costly to be endured. Julie was allowed to find her own path, and as rocky as that was, it was a singularly precious gift.

When children are raised by loving, caring parents, when brothers and sisters show no signs of illness, when expectations for success are unspoken, it can be harder to be the "broken one" than it is for those of us whose homes were hell. One survivor from a middle-class family explained it this way: you know what you've lost. It is impossible not to compare yourself unfavourably with your siblings and to blame yourself for being weak, lazy, or foolish. There is, after all, no one else to blame. You can easily be stuck in the "Why me's?" and feel your life has been stolen from you. Too many of us stop here, and never really get beyond self-pity and self-hate.

*   *   *

Carol Janzen* has been able to move beyond those self-defeating barriers with the help of her family doctor, but not all her medical support has been so caring. Her doctor phoned me last

---

* Carol Janzen is a pseudonym. She asked not to be identified, the only contributor to this book who did so.

year, having run into roadblocks with the psychiatrists at the hospital. The doctor was concerned that Carol was on so much medication she was unable to function, and she was having no luck making that point with the shrinks.

"They're treating her like a chronic, and she's not."

The doctor persisted, making more calls, advocating for her patient, and meeting some success. This is Carol's story.

Carol had been under a lot of stress. She hadn't slept well for a few nights and she'd been depressed for a while. She'd recently separated from her husband, was working, taking three university courses, and raising two children on her own. With no real choice, she pushed through her fatigue, until the morning the ground opened under her feet.

She listened carefully to the voices in her head—it was as though she'd tuned into a radio program featuring her friends and family. They were confessing, one after another, to terrible crimes—the murder of her children. She sensed another presence, one she called her spiritual guru, who wanted to help her know the truth and warn her. She wandered aimlessly through the Mississauga campus of the University of Toronto, where she lived in student housing. Frightened and vulnerable, Carol stopped every few minutes to crouch down, trying to breathe great gasping breaths that failed to calm her.

She knew they were coming for her, too. When she spotted her father's car hunting her, she wanted to run, to escape. But the campus cops pulled up, with someone from health services, and they took her into a building where she was left alone in a small room. There was a noise of something clicking on, of air starting to flow, and she thought, "They're going to gas me." Carol was all fear now. Someone came in with a needle. She backed away, recognizing danger. Security men escorted her upstairs to the psychiatric ward. It was a hospital she was in, or so they said. They left her in a bubble room, with nothing but a foam mattress. When someone appeared who said she was a nurse, Carol felt a little safer and let her inject her with Haldol.

The next morning, she awoke feeling very stiff and very confused. She met with a psychiatrist who told her she'd had a psychotic break.

"I had some difficulty believing him. You don't feel quite sure. And just the thought of it . . . I depended so much on being able to think. How could I function without being able to process things, not knowing reality from hallucinations? Of course, I couldn't verbalize that to them."

They kept her two weeks, and then released her with a prescription and a psychiatric referral. They also gave her the first of three diagnoses: unipolar depression with psychosis. All this was very new and frightening. Although she'd always made friends easily and had a stable home and school life, she suddenly began to isolate herself and to cry frequently.

"I didn't know what was wrong. Everything was black. I felt like I was stuck at the bottom of a well."

Carol had only had one previous experience with the mental health system. At the age of fourteen, just wanting things to be over, wanting the pain to go away, she overdosed on aspirins.

They sent her to a shrink after that, but she only went once. He was busy on the phone making plans to play golf. She never went back to him. She felt a bit exposed after that episode, as if a certain side of her had been revealed, and for a while she felt watched on and off. She had hoped, though, that it would all fade away in time.

Until this episode.

• • •

For Dan, Julie, and Carol, their expectations, ambitions, and need for acceptance had suffered irreparable damage in spite of safe havens at home. There were no bad childhoods, no bad parents, no bad blood. They felt defective and had hard feelings to live with, hard feelings to express.

Things started to go wrong very early for Dan and Julie. It was as though they'd been singled out for rough treatment by some malevolent force. Children often take on more responsibility and guilt than they should ever have to carry, for not being good enough, strong enough. Feeling like a failure even before the onslaught of puberty is not an indicator of a mentally healthy human being.

What happened to Dan at school happens to many mental health patients. They are ridiculed, labelled, and ostracized. There is nothing worse for a kid who desperately craves acceptance. Julie's difference was painful, trapped as she was by ritualistic behaviour that she felt she needed to follow to keep herself and her family safe, although it probably annoyed her siblings. Going for help just brought more negative judgments. Views of self are easily distorted by teachers and helpers, some of whom should not be in positions of trust. I'm sure Dan's teachers and Julie's first shrink did not give another thought to the children they hurt. For Julie and Carol especially, what was happening to them was profoundly frightening, but it didn't compare to the fear, pain, and loss that awaited them once they sought some professional help.

PART TWO

Going in
for Repairs

4.

Hospital:
The Last
Resort

*I quickly learned the basic rules of survival on a psychiatric
ward. Keep your mouth shut. Keep your head down. Take the
medications. Don't make waves.*
— Allan Strong

Sometimes parents wait on the hard chairs in little protective
huddles. At the end of their rope, they know how bizarre and
scary their child's behaviour has become, and they want help.
The hospital is their last hope—the hospital with professional
mental health workers who can diagnosis and medicate and
perhaps return to them the child they know. "Keep him till he's
fixed, can't you?" they ask, expecting much more than is possible.
"We can't cope with him anymore."

But mostly we go by ourselves.

I can understand why Laurie Hall preferred to be carried in by cops, struggling to break free all the while saying: Don't think I want to be in your stupid hospital! Don't think I'm asking you for anything! And I can understand why Allan Strong would go into hospital with his head hanging down, with no fight left in him, even though he knew what was waiting for him: "I quickly learned the basic rules of survival on a psychiatric ward. Keep your mouth shut. Keep your head down. Take the medications. Don't make waves."

As mental health patients, we are fearful of being admitted, and fearful of being sent away. In the midst of this conflict, we lose the art of speech. But because our pain consumes us, we feel it flashes in neon on our foreheads, that everyone knows—especially the health care workers whose business it is to know.

Getting past the gatekeepers in emergency is the first challenge. This involves a great deal of sitting and waiting, looking whole and unhurt amid the carnage of broken bones and bleeding bullet holes, among the stretchers of accident and heart attack victims. First though, we have to find a nurse to tell her—desperately hoping no one overhears—that we need to see the psychiatrist. This often meets with signs of exasperation, indifference, or wariness, with undertones of "Can't you see we have real suffering to deal with here?"

For hours we sit ambivalent, frightened, shunned, certain everyone knows—in the absence of those open wounds—that we're mentally ill. If we've been admitted before, we know the limits and boredom and judgments that await us, and it is harder still. But it's all there is—the only protection on offer.

A big part of us fears that if we're sent away, deemed not crazy enough to warrant one of the few beds still open, it will spell the end. It will be a sign that no one gives a damn and that no one believes how tenuous our hold on life is.

It's not our most rational time.

If we survive the wait, we're examined next by a medical doctor and talked to a little if he or she is nice, and then we wait again. Our pain, our need to be taken seriously, our psychiatric history, our broken selves are about to be judged by experts. This time we sit on a bed shrouded for some illusion of privacy, but of course we can hear moans and groans, questions and answers from beds stretching away on both sides. The words crowd in our heads, all jumbled together, but we cannot speak. Sometimes we can tell right away that we're done for by the impatience on the psychiatrist's face, by his abrupt, cursory questions, as though we're malingering, wasting his time, robbing him of his sleep. Those of us accustomed to not being heard, to not being valued, develop a special vulnerability to the signs that it's happening again. We retreat into silence.

The stories that follow describe how Barry, Laurie, and Julie fared in the sanctuary of the hospital.

*   *   *

Six or seven times during the month since his impromptu "class lecture," Barry D'Costa went to the emergency department of the hospital to ask for something to help him sleep. He would be seen briefly by a crisis worker and given a sedative that he had to take right there, and then he would be sent home by taxi. (You'd think, since he showed up again and again, they might have wondered what else was going on in his life and in his head.) Barry didn't trust them and that didn't help. He couldn't articulate what was keeping him awake days and nights at a time, increasing his fragility, his delusions, and his despair. (Barry's distrust of words is shared by many of us. We know their inadequacy, and we know that once the words are spoken, they can be turned against us and twisted like everything else.)

"Words betray what we have in our heads. The receiver hears something else, and that concerns me a lot. It misconstrues what you mean and therefore who you are as a person. Now I always say, 'Correct me if I'm wrong.' I really wish they'd checked in with me, and asked me if they were hearing what I was saying."

Restless and pacing at home, Barry decided to go to emergency once again.

There was a long wait this time. The crisis worker, who usually came quite quickly, still hadn't arrived. Barry was "exhausted beyond exhaustion," and, without conscious intent, he picked up a sharp blade that had been left with other surgical equipment on a nearby metal table. He started cutting at his wrists. As sad as he was, he remembers feeling quite peaceful as the blood started to flow. Everything got pretty quiet around him. He saw a nurse in front of him, almost as if in a dream, and realized she was trying to speak to him. The sound was calm, but her eyes were really big, as if she'd been badly frightened. Everything seemed to be flying around him—people were running. Barry couldn't respond to the nurse. He couldn't hear anything anymore, but he could sense the frenzy of activity.

At some point they brought in a uniformed security guard. In Barry's tortured mind, the Nazis he feared had finally arrived, setting off extreme panic in him. He was up and running, tripping over a bucket of soapy water, and spilling it. He lay there, watching his blood merge with the puddle, turning everything red.

Staff lifted him up, put him on a stretcher, and moved towards him with a needle. When he awoke, Barry couldn't move his body. He thought he was paralyzed. Heart-stopping minutes later, he realized he was strapped to the bed by his arms and legs and chest. He tried to call out, but his mouth wasn't working and the words weren't coming. The medication they'd shot him up with left him as rigid as a block of wood. A nurse finally came, untied the restraints, and gave him water, which he gulped back to relieve the extreme dryness in his throat. His sister and her boyfriend, the young teaching assistant she would later marry, came to see him that afternoon. At some point, his sister asked where he'd left his car. He kept trying to get the words out, and finally could only yell, "It!" All the muscles in his throat constricted and he couldn't breathe. He was injected with a drug to ease the side effects of the first shot.

He kept drinking water, but he couldn't pee. This went on for three days before he was subjected to the painful experience of a catheter. His father came by, briefly, uncomfortably. (Barry was the first person in his family to go to the nuthouse, his extended family was quick to say: he didn't get it from us.) Sometimes his dad would bring the youngest daughter, and Barry would always try to be at his best, to laugh and joke—to protect her from knowing. All the while, he was learning about the ward, the staff, and the limits of sanctuary.

He says he heard a female patient screaming for help, endlessly banging on the door of her isolation room. He knew staff could hear her too, and yet they weren't responding. A human being in trouble shouldn't be ignored he felt, so he did what's known as the "Thorazine shuffle" to her locked door to see what he could do to comfort her. A male nurse pulled him away, telling him he had no business there.

"What could I do? If I'd persisted, they would have thrown me into isolation, or worse—discharged me."

· · · ·

It is always there as a last resort, until that first admission—a place that means safety, sanctuary, though there is a price to pay. Admission to a psychiatric ward means you are a psychiatric patient, and that label will stick with you always. It defines how people will see you from then on.

Mental patient.

At first, it can be such a relief to finally get there: letting go of the struggle to keep above rising water, handing oneself over, turning oneself in. But what we see around us—the way other patients are treated and the way staff interact with us—clearly shows the limits of this sanctuary, the limits of intervention. We can feel as powerless here as we did at home, in the face of another kind of violence—one rooted in indifference. Or so it appears when someone screams for help and no one comes.

It could be you in that room.

Barry did not find much help there, not this time, and not the next time. He did want to feel better, more in control, but to get there he would have to trust people who didn't seem worthy of that trust. At one point during his confinements, he heard that there was to be an open house at a survivor self-help group. Someone was going to make a presentation about the event to the "discharge group" (people who were getting ready to leave the hospital). Though Barry wasn't up for discharge, he could get a pass to go outside, so he went to the open house and met the survivors. In some ways, it was like going home, only a better home than he'd known. He realized he could be happy working with these people. He could find challenge and comfort in the survivor community.

·   ·   ·

Although Barry could see a positive way to survive as an ex-psychiatric patient, not everyone is as hopeful. Once a patient has seriously considered suicide, once those first steps have been taken to carry it out, it can become the option of choice for all difficult times, and the only hope of escaping the pain. It's as if you start a drug career by smoking crack, going straight to the hard drugs, and skip the pot stage.

I find it telling that part of the training for young suicide bombers is to have them get used to the idea of death by sleeping alone in cemeteries. Though survivors don't go quite that far, we do lose the fear of dying by cradling thoughts of release deep within, images of some dark knight riding to our rescue, slaying the dragons of life that consume us. We learn quickly that needing help only makes us more vulnerable, more exposed to more hurt. It leaves us angry and raging that we've set ourselves up once again for rejection, that we've enabled people to do it to us again.

We want to kill that need in ourselves, to punish that need.

•   •   •   •

Laurie Hall had still not found a way to deal with her anger and guilt—anger at the father who had made her into his punching bag and guilt about the siblings she'd left behind.

"I was trying to coast without any coping skills."

They'd tried giving her four-point restraints on a PRN (patient requests nurse) basis to control her rage.

"Sometimes I hated it; sometimes I needed it. It was better than throwing furniture, though it didn't necessarily feel that way. Throwing furniture—at walls, not people—made me feel powerful, stronger, able to put some of my anger out there."

Even today, Laurie prefers winter because she can bulk up with layers of clothes and be bigger than she is, feel more powerful.

The last time she had been discharged, the hospital pharmacy gave her a month's worth of all her medications: "I felt kind of like they were saying 'Go ahead, do it,' so I did." She took everything they'd given her, including pills to lower blood pressure, which is what caused lasting damage to her bowel.

After that, Laurie woke up in a hospital bed with a tube down her throat, another down her nose, a "kind of tap in my neck," more tubes running in both of her arms, and, just to complete the horrific picture, a big tube coming out of her stomach. Lying there, she had a vague memory of the lights and voices in the emergency ward, of her belly all swollen and hurting "like period cramps," of a bearded man with a surgeon's cap listening to her stomach with a stethoscope saying in concerned tones, "No bowel sounds."

The doctors called her parents. Half her bowel had been removed, pneumonia had set in, and death appeared to be imminent. Her parents said they wouldn't be able to come until next week. That was an epiphany for Laurie.

She realized in a moment of stunning clarity that most of her actions in the past few years had been unconscious attempts to get her parents to show they cared. Now that she knew this was never going to happen, she stopped hoping, stopped expecting. Instead of this brutal awareness being the final blow, it was strangely liberating. Gradually, she began to realize that the hospital wasn't going to hand her a cure either.

I can almost see Laurie wandering around the ward, looking under tables and chairs, staring at the doctors, nurses, and patients, searching for a cure that simply wasn't there. She must have asked herself why she kept returning, only to be rebuffed, overmedicated, and tied down.

"Sitting there in a Johnny shirt, day after day, nothing going on, no real therapy, it was almost worse than being outside."

It's a scary decision never to go back, and it took Laurie quite a while to give up on the promise of a cure. But when she finally looked to herself to make life valuable, she was firmly planted on the road to recovery.

We have to learn to make the system work for us, not against us, to hang in until we find someone—and they are out there—who can see and hear us. I have heard, at different times, two hospital administrators say that cleaning and kitchen staff have forged better relationships with in-patients than the doctors and nurses on-site have. Unencumbered by knowledge of diagnoses, symptoms, and background, and unable to prescribe medications, restraints, and time-outs, the support staff react as people should to anyone in pain—with caring, conversation, and support.

Why do we collude with gatekeepers in institutions that turn us away when we finally ask for help? I'm not sure why, underneath our tough, "who gives a damn" exteriors, we remain so raw and sensitive to rejection, criticism, and attitude. Our calluses are skin deep, but they are more visible than the needs we feel and are fearful to express.

*   *   *

Julie Flatt, in spite of the horror stories she'd heard as a child and of her fear of being institutionalized, was eventually admitted to hospital. The inappropriately named "daycare" program she attended brought to mind toddlers and mid-afternoon naps, rather than adults with mental illnesses who needed structure and watching. Julie found it very scary. She didn't want anything to do with the nurses, and the "pressure to talk in 'therapy circles' while staff sat silent, letting us know that we should initiate discussion, was a big joke."

"They had all the control. I remember them making me lie on the floor in the dark, no blankets, with thirty other mental patients, listening to my breathing, which I was sure was too loud. It was supposed to teach us how to relax! It was so uncomfortable. I lost all confidence from being in hospital, learning to be even more skeptical of services, seeing in them another part of the loss of control, when I'd already lost my mind."

Julie never warmed to the staff there or at the other places she was destined to go.

"I kept them at bay, though I learned to act as if I liked them, to get by. I resented them for, I guess, doing their jobs. It was the authoritarian role: here I was 'letting my mind go,' and they were the people you went to, to get yourself propped up again. People like that who see people like me and worse and who don't cry every night—they can't be compassionate. They hadn't been anywhere near where I was; they just saw a collection of clinical symptoms. Nothing was touching them; they had no great gaps in their work history. The way professionals are taught tells them nothing about us. To me, they were in the judgment seat, they could say 'assert yourself' and teach me things like that, but they didn't get how hard things hurt. I didn't want to be there, didn't want to be considered mentally ill. The old image of 'locked up in the attic,' that interpretation was still there, and I didn't want to be in a place that said I was less than other people."

Julie was singularly unlucky in the staff she encountered. No one broke through and related person-to-person, rather than staff-to-patient.

Barry D'Costa had also attended day treatment programs between hospital in-patient stays: "I was glad when they finally kicked me out, otherwise I would have quietly, privately done myself in. Nurses grouping us together, getting us to spill our guts in what felt like a public violation. Occupational therapists telling us how to make toast."

For me, it was the endless games of volleyball. Medicated people made spastic efforts to hit a ball over a net, shuffling around the gym, while the staff's forced cheerful banter tried to inject some enthusiasm. It felt like an obscenity to those trapped inside their heads—playing children's games while so many big questions remained unanswered, unaddressed.

How do I live with how I feel?

How do I go back to work when I can barely function?

How can I get back to myself?

Staff and patients seem so far apart, from two different worlds. Staff have the keys; they have all the control; they make all the decisions—life and death decisions. Who goes, who stays, who gets put in those scary little rooms, who gets injected with chemical restraints—it's all based on how they interpret you, on who they think you are.

We're judging them too, but our judgment has no power. We watch them as they move about the ward looking self-assured and unaffected by the misery around them. Patients have a built-in radar that tells them quickly, unequivocally, who gives a damn and who's just putting in time. We want those indifferent staff members to know we're on to them, that we're not fooled when they apply a thin mask of concerned interest, talking just long enough to have something to put in the chart for that shift. It's a matter of self-respect for us.

It never occurred to me that they could be fearful of approaching us, fearful of being rejected, of having their feelings bruised. During my last hospitalization, a nurse dared to tell me, after I'd dismissed her efforts to engage me, how hard it was to talk to me, how she had to screw up her courage to even try.

It was a revelation.

Underneath all that authority, they were human beings who could be hurt and who could feel rejected. They could react honestly, rather than professionally. Many of us aren't afforded that knowledge.

Barry told me a story about a patient who was being discharged from the ward. She cursed and stormed at a particular nurse on her way out, calling her every name in the book before the doors closed behind her. He told it from the perspective of the patient, who was getting her own back, and he was surprised when I asked him how the nurse had felt. He'd never thought about it, never considered that this staff person might have been affected by the verbal assault.

A revelation for him too.

With every one of my hospital admissions except one, that one being to the provincial hospital, there was a nurse who was real. These nurses broke the rules in one way or another, and trusted me with glimpses of who they were. They dared to be more than one-dimensional "keepers"; they dared to be human. They were so much more effective than the ones who simply enforced the rules and handed out medications, hiding behind their roles. They closed the gap between patient and nurse, and reminded me that we were more than illnesses. They could see us beneath symptoms and behaviours, even value us.

Those moments, those staff, were the sanctuary we sought.

5.

My Confinement

Few of us ever feel ready to leave. Few of us ever feel fixed.
        —Pat Capponi

I could not seem to do without it.

From a distressed distance, it always looked more comforting than its actuality. Besides, it was the only game in town. On the hospital ward, after my pockets were emptied of anything potentially dangerous or intoxicating, after I had traded my street clothes for a Johnny shirt and my shoes for paper slippers, after I had no more control over my life: I was accepted as a mental patient.

Hospital admittance can be a validation, especially if relatives and friends have nagged us to pull up our socks, to get some backbone, to stop being self-indulgent slugs. It reminds me of the story of the lifelong hypochondriac who had the epitaph "I Told You I Was Sick" carved on his gravestone.

There can be a great relief in handing yourself over to be fixed. There's no longer a solitary, wearisome, daily struggle. There's no longer a struggle at all: you slip into a passive role in the face of all the expertise that surrounds you and conspires to keep you safe, make you well.

And you wait, and you wait, and you wait some more, for the experts to fix you.

Wards are often deadly boring places to be, but boredom is interspersed with moments of high drama—a suicide attempt, an assault, a new admission screaming out her psychosis from a locked room—all are reminders of your own reality in a place where reality is kept at bay. You learn quickly how small you are in the face of your illness—how helpless, needy, and lost.

You become dependent and institutionalized, just as a prisoner does. All responsibility is removed from you: when to shower, when to eat, when to go to bed, when to get up, when to take the pills, when to talk to the nurse and doctor, when to go to group. Every behaviour is deemed to be outside your control, and so control must be applied externally—by an injection, a tie-down, a suicide watch.

You learn powerlessness in a place where you have no power at all. Others decide about your life and future, in your best interests, of course—judgments based on their narrow interpretations of who you are (diagnosis and prognosis) and what you need (from the pharmaceutical cornucopia), and there is no appeal to a higher court.

The first time I ran away from home to a psychiatric hospital, I didn't feel like a crazy person, though I knew for sure everyone else on the ward was. I watched with a mixture of suspicion and deep caution, expecting them to go off like grenades if I said or did the wrong thing.

I spent a lot of time in my room, hiding. I was often disturbed through the long stretches of night by nurses shining bright flashlights in my eyes. I was awakened early to the first question of the day: Did your bowels move? and to the rumbling of the breakfast carts as they were pushed through the swinging doors by orderlies. Taking a tray and keeping my head down, I tried to find a safe place to sit (harder than it sounds in the crowded dayroom). Medication calls and straggling lineups, ward meetings, occupational therapy, one-on-one meetings with the psychiatrist, the lunch cart, the supper cart, the deadly evening hours—I hated it all.

And then Bo emerged from his darkened room. His overdose of the dangerous street drug belladonna and his subsequent acute photosensitivity had meant weeks of isolation—curtains drawn, lights kept off.

For me, Bo was a breath of fresh air in this stifling environment. He was gentle and funny, and he pretty much embodied the hippie movement with his long hair, John Lennon glasses, torn jeans, and odd ambition to build his own plane. He laughed, hell, he giggled, a bubbling up of reservoirs of humour in one skinny guy. He dramatically altered the hospital experience for me: madness could be fun, liberating even, and occasionally exhilarating.

Laughter had never really been a part of me before. It was the most important "life skill" I learned during my five-month stay.

We became partners in mischief during daring daylight and midnight escapades when we were faster than the alarms on the crash bar door. We tripped down the stairs and out the front doors before aging security guards could catch us. Smoking dope in the bathrooms or on the surrounding property, spitting out medications after pretending to swallow them, liberating the caged "therapeutic canary," we bedevilled the staff and even the psychiatrist who liked us both.

Bo taught me to play ping-pong and pool. He was a much better role model for madness than the weepy, defeated, middle-class women who'd been turned in by disgruntled husbands or the shambling, overmedicated, pyjama-clad men who didn't know where they were. His ability to see the absurd, to undermine the governing regime, and to question the assumptions about our mental illness served us both well.

In Bo's presence, I could withstand what sometimes seemed absurdly like a Finishing School regime on the ward, where nurses and doctors would despair of my jeans and straight hair, of my unladylike behaviour and profane language that would never win me a husband, children, and a home in the suburbs.

I could forget the gnawing reality that I had nowhere to go if and when I left this place. I was eighteen, a runaway, with no resources, no home, and no future that I could envision. All I owned were the clothes on my back and this new label that seemed to be tattooed on my forehead: mental patient.

When Bo was discharged a month or two before me, it seemed like the lights dimmed. The dull, everyday routine began to chafe more. Decisions had to be made—I couldn't stay here forever.

In the sixties and early seventies, when I was coming into consciousness, a man's home was still his castle, and his wife and children were his to do with as he pleased. Education for girls: that was just something to fall back on if and when the marriage didn't work out. Bell Telephone and Sun Life were touted as the best places to go after graduation—jobs for twenty years to life, pension plans, and homes in all-white neighbourhoods. Gays were deep in the closet; crazy people were in their straitjackets; natives were on their reserves; and unhappy women were on Valium.

But I had read Kafka, Sartre, Salinger, Dostoyevsky, and Steinbeck—counterpoints to Hula Hoops, Lawrence Welk, Charlton Heston, Howdy Doody, Maggie Muggins, Leave It to Beaver, The Honeymooners, *and endless World War II documentaries. I had listened to Bob Dylan and folk music. I knew about George Wallace and dead little black girls in a bombed-out church, nuclear proliferation, and planetary death.*

Though the hippie movement brought me great comfort (my worldview and jeans were finally in style), it did not break through to the hospitals, those arbiters of normalcy, or to a middle class for whom Father Knows Best *still had some resonance.*

I was still hugely susceptible to negative judgments, unaware that my choices and my "lifestyle" threatened those with a heavy investment in the status quo.

Psychiatrists comfortably ensconced on the top rungs of their professional ladder preferred not to consider any other reality than the one they were educated to administer. Nurses in their makeup and carefully styled hair, in their showcase dresses,

*nylons, and heels, in their wholehearted embrace of their roles
and realities, had every reason to believe that society was fine just
as it was.*

*My rejection of this worldview questioned their choices and
ambitions, and therefore in their opinion had to have some pathological base that required medication, therapy, and fixing.*

*Still, I understood that no matter how I'd arrived at my way of
thinking and seeing, it was as valid and real (perhaps more so, I'd
defiantly tell myself) as theirs, and deep, deep down I knew that it
required courage and suffering to maintain that vision. If anyone
had asked, I might have said I needed help holding on to that
darker reality I had experienced and known. I needed a way to
deal with the pain I felt and the fear that I had that I had perhaps
moved so far from the mainstream there was no going back. Not
that I'd ever really been conventional, but those authorities scared
me with their insistence that if I didn't change now the way they
prescribed, it would soon be too late. I'd be so far gone along a
separate path that my destruction would be inevitable.*

*The few times I stumbled over words trying to express all this—
before I completely gave up trying to reach them—I was accused of
"intellectualizing" my problems. Spiritual angst didn't seem to
exist outside the realm of delusion; seeking and sensing a greater
purpose than what they laid out as the greatest good was clear
evidence to them of my psychosis. It was very silencing.*

*There was some change for the better during my five-month stay
at the hospital: I wasn't crying all the time—I'd hated that part of
this craziness thing. Crying always felt like a bitter defeat, a giving*

in. My father had always hit us, kicked us, and punched us until we cried.

I was still mostly composed of sadness. I still leapt out of my skin at every loud noise, harsh voice, dropped fork, and ring of the patients' payphone. I would still hunch over my meal tray, expecting eruptions from the tables near me, struggling to swallow every bland mouthful.

I hadn't found any sense here of my place in the world or any great enthusiasm for searching it out. After Bo left, I would take myself over to the housing construction site we had once explored together on our AWOL expeditions, to the fresh smell of sawdust and the sucking sound of mud underfoot, but it wasn't the same. I remember leaving the wooden frame building and standing alone on the sidewalk of the barren suburb, staring into a distance that was as bleak as my thoughts. Remember this, I demanded of myself. Remember this fear, this uncertainty. Come back to this time and have something to say about who you've become, what you've accomplished. It was a desperately optimistic moment, a weary, dreadful half-prayer, half-commitment to life.

Towards the end of my stay, Robert Kennedy was assassinated. I remember all of us crazy people being gathered up for an impromptu ward meeting. The announcement was made by the reigning psychiatrist, who was clearly shaken. We were invited to speak about what we were feeling. A long moment of unbroken silence followed as we sat there in our cushioned medicated states, absorbed in our own lives, in our own pain, so that the tragic fate of another Kennedy had no resonance. I watched the staff and understood at some level that this meeting wasn't about our needs or reactions, it was about their pain, their shock at their world shattering, their need for reassurance. They seemed almost angry when the silence went on so long they had to release us from that artificial "therapeutic" circle. They had to deal with their own heads and hearts and their fears as people rather than as professionals.

As for me, decisions were made about my future. I would not be sent back home, but to Toronto to join my older sister, Terry, who was teaching in an elementary school there.

I got a job at a department store and tried to fit in.

It was hopeless, and I lost ground the way I still do when trying to be something I'm not.

I couldn't breathe in the airless atmosphere, in the colourless sameness of every day—a paycheque wasn't enough to compensate for losing my soul.

     •   •   •

After that first one, there were six more admissions to three different hospitals.

There was nothing I could point to on the wards that was worth returning to. I could not say with any confidence: This will make me better; this will keep me safer. But I knew with absolute certainty that left on my own, I would die. I came back to the deadening routine of occupational therapy and group meetings— to those uncomfortable one-on-one sessions with the (usually) authoritarian psychiatrist and to the rigid structure of when to get up, when to eat, when to go back to bed, when to take the pills, when to shower.

I was surrounded by walking, sometimes talking, bundles of misery and pain. You breathe that atmosphere in; it gets in your blood. If part of the problems you had came from feeling too much, the hospital environment could be tortuous.

In the hospitals, young people, casualties of the drug culture, were taking up more beds. LSD and speed could fracture the minds of the unsuspecting, sending them spinning into psychosis, sometimes never to return. Staff must have felt besieged by this raucous, questioning group that didn't respond well to power and control and didn't see conformity and productivity as the greatest good.

The world was changing and this was just the beginning: Kent State, Vietnam, Nixon, Watergate, there was even wife-swapping and prostitution in the chaste suburbs. So many young people rejected the hypocrisy and pretence that all was well. They couldn't all be mentally ill.

Much later, I was on another ward when Trudeau declared the War Measures Act and armed Canadian troops occupied the streets of Montreal. Kidnapped British trade commissioner James Cross was flown to our hospital after his release by the FLQ. Soldiers blocked every entrance. The crazier it got out there as politicians, radicals, and police clashed, the more sense our pain made. But we were the ones viewed as insane. We were the ones who needed watching, medicating, and restraining. I was starting to learn, if not yet accept, that reality can't be cured; it can be changed maybe, but not cured.

This is why I came to see hospitalization as a betrayal of self. Admittance to hospital would come when the world as I knew it, saw it, and experienced it, wore me down, drove me mad, when I wanted to escape, blind myself, see through their eyes, accept their delusions in place of my reality. My way of seeing the world, my awareness of the violence, hatred, prejudice, lies, hypocrisy, and corruption left me depressed and suicidal—there was no cure for what was out there.

All this conspired against accepting the patient "role." I played out my inner turmoil and self-hate with cutting, slashing, and burning—building a file that would eventually label me as chronic and send me from the civility of a middle-class psychiatric ward to the dead end of a provincial hospital.

. . .

Few of us ever feel ready to leave. Few of us ever feel fixed. We must return to lives that we ran from in the first place, and nothing's really changed. We're not stronger. We haven't figured out why we do things that get us into trouble.

And so we go back.

As long as they keep re-admitting us, in spite of our ambivalence about life on the ward, there is hope that we won't have to always feel and live this way, that this time they might get it right. It's as optimistic as we get. But for the psychiatrists, this is evidence of chronicity and dependence. As our files thicken, their patience thins.

• • •

The Douglas Hospital a.k.a. the Verdun.

A sprawling collection of buildings called pavilions back then, this old hospital was filled with the misery and loss of thousands of men and women who'd come through the doors and never left, not standing anyway. It's where they sent you when the doctors and nurses got tired of you not getting better, where the chronic label was slapped on your forehead, and where containment seemed the only goal.

People, normal people in the surrounding communities, whispered about the place, skirted it, and made whistling-in-the-dark jokes about the inmates. This place wasn't for the delicate, middle-class patient crumbling under stress. This was the big time. This was where time stopped.

Mental illness looked more like a disease of the body here, as though a plague had left the same physical effects on everyone it touched: jerky movements, facial tics and spasms, enlarged tongues, and drool pooled at the corners of the mouth. Worse for me, the bedrooms were locked during the dayshift, so there was no retreat from the sights and sounds, the screams and howls, and the imminent threats all around. I don't remember one name or one person from my long months there. Boredom and fear played off against each other. There was no safety, not even a pretence of therapy, and no expectation of getting better or getting out.

The nurses and orderlies seemed as frightened as me, protected in their glass-walled stations. It was clear they didn't enjoy their jobs, more custodial than medical, and they resented how they had to earn their living. They understood the patients they sought to control even less than I did. We were the untouchables; they were the unapproachable guardians of society.

I didn't wonder what had sent these men and women patients tumbling over the edge. Their humanity was obscured, almost erased, by decades of confinement, powerful and brutal antipsychotics, acute loneliness, and loss. I didn't draw an easy breath the whole time I was in that particular corner of hell.

And when I was finally released, I fled to Toronto, faraway from echoes of unrestrained madness. Or so I thought. But there was another stay on another ward, a more civil and genteel ward, and then finally a move to the Parkdale boarding home. Once again, I would encounter men and women from provincial madhouses, from the Verduns of Ontario—Whitby, Lakeshore, and Queen Street. In that boarding home, however, I was eventually able to get past the frightening exteriors to the humanity within.

•   •   •   •

The current response to the pain of those labelled mentally ill is to block up all the exits— the bridges, overpasses, and subways— where people try to commit suicide. This is easier than improving the quality of their desperate lives. Society seeks to confine those brought to the edge, to protect them from themselves, but there is little in place to guard us from these protectors. In the hospital, staff remove "dangerous" belongings and reduce patients' identity to narrow plastic wrist bracelets. It can feel more like being in a prison than a hospital.

It wasn't so very long ago that men and women who were physically ill refused to go into hospital. They understood that of those who went in, few came out. To spend their last days in a crowded ward with tired nursing staff was not a dignified end. The limits of medicine and medical intervention were clearer then—before the term *modern medicine* suggested that almost everything could be cured.

Many psychiatric patients have learned that hospitals are not appropriate places to treat the pain of the mentally ill. The word *hospital* suggests pathology and science, and that expertise and medicine will be brought to bear on mental disease. There isn't much room in all this bustling professionalism for simple humanity and person-to-person caring.

The Gerstein Centre in Toronto is an alternative to hospitalization. When Dr. Reva Gerstein was appointed by then-Toronto-Mayor Art Eggleton to serve as the Mayor's Action Task Force on Discharged Psychiatric Patients, she asked if I would be on her advisory committee. We held hearings at city hall and in the Parkdale drop-in where I worked, so that ex-patients could speak with us directly. One concrete result was the establishment of the Gerstein Centre for those experiencing psychosocial crisis. While it was being developed, there was great concern in government circles that there would not be any experts (psychiatrists, social workers, and nurses) on staff. Doctors and family groups thought it foolhardy and dangerous not to focus on diagnosis, prognosis, and medications. But Dr. Gerstein listened to us as survivors when we expressed our fears of being hospitalized and of losing control in our treatment. She heard how we needed a place that would respect our whole beings and our personal struggles for autonomy.

The hiring committee, of which I was a member, looked for people who exuded warmth rather than expertise and who would not resort to the power imbalances so common in psychiatric hospitals. We wanted people who would help the clients define their own needs, rather than health care workers who would impose their own solutions and then blame the client when those solutions didn't work.

When Barry D'Costa found himself slipping, he hesitatingly checked in to the Gerstein Centre. One night he was working on some papers, playing catch-up with work, and he felt the presence of a staff person behind him. It was getting late, and he fully expected to be told to go to bed—tired hospital nurses would always want their patients sleeping on schedule. He was surprised and pleased when the staff member leaned over and plugged in a lamp so that he could see better. Barry realized he could leave for work in the morning and return in the evening, like a real person. He wasn't required to give up everything he had achieved in his working life to get some help.

The staff at the Gerstein do not filter everything through diagnosis, so the effects of poor housing, lack of community and opportunity, and poverty can be assessed as well as mental health. Unlike large institutions that foster dependence and alienation, small, homelike places such as the Gerstein Centre speak to the real needs of the whole person. And if people like ourselves are employed there, too, we will learn that there is a way to thrive, even with a mental illness.

* * *

Over time, staff from Toronto's Queen Street Mental Health Centre—known as the "bin"—became human beings to me, engaged in their own struggles. [I had never been a patient there.] They were not cardboard cutouts with keys. I socialized with them, and even dated some of them, while working at Parc. I had only known the world of the patient; my perspective was widened, and my eyes fully opened. I knew now there were no easy answers that they kept from us, no secret knowledge, no magic cure that they held just out of reach.

There was a lot of drinking and partying as people who worked at the bin tried to relieve the tension of their jobs, their working environment, and their marriages. Staff were dealing or not dealing with their own feelings of disempowerment and resentment, sparked by supervisors and government policies that sometimes seemed crazier than their patients.

And when they lost a patient to suicide, a far too common event, it would rock them as badly as it rocked me; but they didn't have the same freedom that I did to speak the truth at the inquests into those deaths. Corralled and controlled by lawyers for the hospital and the ministry, these employees would sit apart from the deceased's family and any survivors present during days and weeks of testimony, fearful of being blamed, of being hung out to dry by their employers.

It was difficult to be friends, even lovers in some instances, with people who were suddenly on the other side, whether they wanted to be or not. But again, it made me aware of the human side of those who'd been our keepers—that they too were vulnerable and even broken in some of the same ways we were. I'd watch them sometimes, in bars and restaurants, listen to their stories and grievances, and wonder why I'd ever thought they "had it all" when it came to sanity and making it in the outside world.

It helped me to speak to staff in ways that would reach those capable of hearing, when conducting "sensitization" sessions with groups of mental health workers from hospitals and agencies. I would talk about increasing their level of job satisfaction by partnering with survivors rather than working on them. I tried to recapture their initial enthusiasm for the work they were involved in and to recognize the ways in which their feelings of powerlessness were passed on to their clients.

It was also empowering to sit on hiring committees, to question prospective staff at places like the Gerstein Centre, the Provincial Patient Advocate Office, and the Ontario Advocacy Commission, and to articulate a common definition of what makes a good staff, and even participate in their training.

Not surprisingly, it was human qualities rather than academic credentials that we looked for. We wanted people who weren't afraid to feel, to reach out, and to care. We wanted people who understood the limits of a textbook education and the medical model. We wanted people with a history of going to bat for their clients.

We wanted people who would help other people, not add to the burden of hurt.

6.

Diagnosis
and
Drugs

Massachusetts, grappling with soaring Medicaid prescription drug costs, will warn doctors about a practice officials say costs millions and may harm some patients: physicians prescribing multiple psychiatric drugs—sometimes as many as seven—to individual patients. . . .

Many psychiatrists see poly-prescribing as part of the art of treating the mentally ill, a sort of improvisational medicine; they know that many expensive new psychiatric drugs—or combinations of them—work for some patients, but they don't know exactly how. And they can't predict which drugs will help which patients. . . .

—Liz Kowalczyk, "State Seeks Psychiatric Drug Cuts," *The Boston Globe,* July 12, 2002

The most radical changes for psychiatric survivors always seem to begin with cost-cutting. Though it's been frequently denied, I am certain that the reason for the rapid, uncontrolled closure of hospital beds (and hospitals) that began in the seventies and continues to this day, was motivated more by economic considerations than by a liberal view that antipsychotic medications now made it possible for patients to return to their communities. And though the consequent lack of planning, loss of housing, and income support have caused unimaginable suffering, at least as survivors we have escaped captivity and the back wards that once entombed us.

Now once again, as the above quote shows, the amount and mix of medications to keep us out of hospital may finally be undergoing scrutiny, thanks to rising costs. The pharmaceutical lobby is very strong, as is the medical system that supports it. There are few champions willing to go up against either of these groups, for fear of being isolated and branded modern-day heretics by the establishment.

Most people's lives are messy and complicated, but this is especially true for psychiatric patients. Poverty, hunger, and boredom wear them down, for instance, and just getting through the day creates huge stress. Not everything can be explained in terms of symptomology. Social exclusion and stigma isolate individuals. Abuse continues to haunt people long after the bruises have faded.

And there's something else. Imagine you were given drugs for indigestion or an ulcer, but you'd actually had a heart attack!

Clearly, the diagnosis has to be accurate for medications to work. Mental health patients realized, however, after talking among themselves, that they have been repeatedly misdiagnosed and given the wrong medications, sometimes for years. What's worse, they usually take the new medications before the old ones are out of their systems. Only a few lucky patients are admitted and watched for negative effects while the changeover occurs.

*   *   *

Barry D'Costa had five hospital admissions, "nailing all the seasons" in the process. His first psychiatrist thought he had simple depression; the second labelled him with manic depression; the third with personality disorder; the fourth with schizophrenia; and the fifth with bipolar disorder and schizophrenia.

"I think they based their diagnosis on observing symptoms that weren't inherent to me, but that were emotional and physical side effects from the rapid change of drugs."

He went through a battery of antipsychotic, antianxiety, and antidepressive pills.

"I had more bottles of pills than cans of vegetables in my apartment. I took the drugs more regularly than I ate my meals."

He endured acute photosensitivity, body rashes, and nightmares, and he was out of sorts physically and emotionally. He felt numb, disconnected, and increasingly irritated, as if he had no real control over his muscles. At the same time, he didn't have enough to eat, he was struggling to pay his rent, and his life was not improving. It would not get better until someone finally referred him to community supports that actually helped him.

·   ·   ·

Laurie Hall had her own collection of labels, a half-dozen or so, with pills connected to every one. She couldn't think and she couldn't problem solve. When she was very frustrated, she'd flush her pills down the toilet. Shortly after that she would get sick, and she'd be told: See what happens when you don't take them!

It was maddening.

One of the benefits of being on morphine—Laurie was in considerable pain from an overdose that almost killed her— was that her psychiatric medications had all been stopped. She was recovering her strength and finding new resolve, when a nurse entered her room with a whole tray of psychiatric medications to swallow. The new Laurie said, "Hold on now. I want to know what each of these is supposed to be for, and what the side effects might be."

Laurie was becoming a survivor.

It's a sad fact that survivors get more information from television ads for brand-name drugs than they do from their counsellors.

·   ·   ·

Since her psychotic breakdown at the University of Toronto, Carol Janzen took the medications prescribed for her, but she found that she could barely function. (Her first diagnosis was schizophrenia; the second was manic depression; and after that, the one that stuck was bipolar with schizo-affective disorder.)

Carol wishes she'd been told soon after her first dramatic incident that it takes a long time to find the right medication. Whenever a medication failed, it seemed a failure on her part. And it didn't help when she was told it was the illness, not the pills, that left her feeling awful, even though dosages or types of chemical intervention would change when she complained, leading her to feel it *was* the medications.

Some pills made her feel as if worms were eating her brain. Lithium spun her off into mania, something she'd never experienced before. Like Barry, she had difficulty with physical movement. She gained seventy pounds during this time.

"Every time I went to the psychiatrist's, it was like putting my head on the chopping block. What would they do to me this time? They kept slamming me with different drugs, different dosages."

She would stare out the window for hours "going psychologically comatose."

If it weren't for her love and sense of responsibility for her children, she might not have been so compliant about taking such a cornucopia of medications. She had to get back to herself and back to them, while she struggled to complete her degree and to work. There were times when she despaired, telling her psychiatrist: "I might as well be dead. My life is over. It's one thing to lose a limb, but not being able to trust your brain!"

Carol is still coming to terms with everything that's happened to her. It would have helped if she had gone through a grieving process to deal with how she feels about her diagnosis and treatment. She hasn't yet had a calm, quiet space to catch up with herself. She was very lucky that her family doctor (and mine), Pauline Pariser, went to bat for her. Pauline became Carol's advocate. It's one thing for the patient to declare that the medications are too heavy, but quite another for a doctor to do so.

"They were treating her like a chronic, and she's not."

Carol had to face the consequences that she could not handle the minimum number of university courses and therefore was no longer eligible for student housing. The man in charge of housing was very decent about allowing her to stay as long as possible, but he was retiring. Finally she had to move, and that was another stressor for her and her family.

And she is second-guessing herself: Perhaps if she hadn't gone to university, all this chaos might never have happened. But she "loves her English courses so much" and she's just four subjects short of getting a degree—a lifelong ambition. It wasn't easy to go back to school and be so visible after her breakdown. Barry solved this by waiting a year to go back, so that he joined a new batch of students who wouldn't have witnessed his full psychotic break. Carol runs into people who know her and who think she must be on her Master's by now.

"It makes me feel like less of a person." But she keeps going. It has been five years since that afternoon when the voices started in her head.

She's bought a dog and that gets her out exercising, tackling the extra weight, clearing her head. Although she's not exactly hopeful, she is making changes to accommodate this disease. She's moving forward.

* * *

There is always so much extra baggage that goes along with mental illness. Each piece can come to seem as if it's part of the illness, to the point where it becomes disproportionately large and beyond our ability to conquer it. When I work with groups of survivors, one of the first things I do is separate out all the different elements that are preying on them, something that psychiatrists rarely do. If everything we feel becomes the mental illness, it becomes overwhelming and beyond our ability to conquer. This is a helpful exercise, because breaking down all the different factors that go into holding us back, into holding us down as surely as four-point restraints, will reduce feelings of helplessness and defeat. We can do something about the separate elements. We can strengthen that original self (and it may well be the first time we've heard that) and we can reduce the impact of the labels that we carry.

In these groups, we talk first about the self, the part of us that was us before we were labelled. I'll ask them about that self, and what it hoped for out of life. The answers are usually the ordinary things that make anyone's life worth living. Then, we talk about the trauma of being diagnosed, and for most that's exactly what it is, a traumatic death sentence. I'll tap people on the shoulder as I move about the room, saying you're the self and you're the label you've been given. They see how the label looms so large that it obscures the self.

Then we discuss the medications. Whether they help or not, there is usually a price to pay for taking them. People talk about the side effects, separating them out from the disease: the inability to concentrate, to read, to sit still or to move; the constant fatigue like being wrapped in layers of heavy cloth; impotence, shaking, sleeping too much or too little. Given all these side effects, it's little wonder that shrinks don't really see what's happening with their clients.

Most survivors are poor, the consequence of being labelled and medicated. Poverty is crushing even when nothing else is going on. Survivors mention shame, depression, stress, hunger, fear, and boredom as features of "simple" poverty—all these consequences of poverty are almost indistinguishable from the mental illness we're supposed to have. Andrew Solomon, in a *New York Times* article (May 6, 2001), draws attention to the suffering of the poor: "But among the indigent, the traumas are so terrible and so frequent, says Jeanne Miranda (associate professor at Georgetown University) that searching for the depressed among them is like checking for emphysema among coal miners."

Then, of course, there's isolation, social stigma, and the gnawing sense of loss. The self pretty much disappears as we seem to become the physical manifestation of mental illness.

*   *   *

There is a vocal minority in the survivor movement that seeks to discourage survivors from taking the medications that are prescribed for them. I see in that the same kind of best-interest thinking and arrogance that we get from the doctors. People have a right to make their own decisions—to choose or not to choose psychiatric drugs. They also have a right to all the information available about the drugs they take. And they should not have to be defensive about deciding to stay on pills.

To Jill Stainsby, this is a sore point.

"My opinion that I can function on medications but not without them is just a truth, to me; to have my perceptions so completely discounted by antipsychiatry survivors is disaffirming. There is a feminist concept regarding stories of abuse, particularly domestic abuse, which is represented by the catchphrase 'believe the woman.' In this case, I find that this element of the movement does not believe me, or many like me, who experience an improved quality of life (in our own critical self-awareness) once medicated. The limitation is theirs."

Take them, don't take them—it's as specious a debate as whether or not mental illness exists. Survivors should understand what they're taking and why. They need to understand the different factors that have gone in to keeping them crazy and work on those things. The more our quality of life improves, the fewer pills we have to take: it's a proven fact.

.   .   .

In the survivor movement, we have a slogan: a home, a job, and a friend. It may surprise the reader that such basic and necessary elements were not always considered part of the needs of the mentally ill. We had to demand that programs provided quality of life, not just maintenance in the community. We did not want to be crowded into boarding houses, targeted by case management teams, and medicated to keep us quiescent and out of the hospital.

Chemical restraints are as effective in the community as the physical four-point restraints that tied us to our hospital beds. There is no question that the medications are not for us, but rather to reassure the rest of society, who are made nervous, fearful, and unhappy by our presence in their midst.

I remember the day I was discharged from St. Michael's hospital. I was getting ready to travel to the boarding home for ex-psychiatric patients, which would be the biggest shock and challenge I would ever face. The head nurse, a nice, caring man whom I quite liked, said to me: "I wish we could have done more for you." How I wished that too. I was leaving the safety of the ward to try life on the outside once again, knowing that I still had no investment in living, no enthusiasm for what lay ahead, and no idea where they were sending me. Even the doctors and nurses didn't know what I was going to. The boarding home was just listed as one of the recommended housing alternatives in whatever manual the social worker had consulted. Three months

and eleven days of expensive care that included constant observation, group therapy, suicide watches, and counselling were all
at risk as I walked out one door and through another: Why had
they bothered?

In the boarding home, there were rooms where three, four,
even five people would try to co-exist, lying on different-sized
beds that were fitted into whatever available space could be
found, through the daylight and evening hours. The only
"personal" possessions most had were endless bottles of pills,
clustered together, some gathering dust, others swallowed faith-
fully—pills for this, that, and the other, sent monthly from the
local drugstore, charged to welfare or to family benefits. No one
who lived there really knew their diagnosis or could pronounce
the names of their meds, never mind understand what they were
supposed to do.

Medications continued to arrive, sometimes for months, after
the death of a tenant, or a disappearance, or an eviction. Often if
a tenant was being difficult or threatening, the landlord would
force him to take someone else's pills in order to subdue him, and
then send him back to his bed.

Sometimes it seemed that was the doctor's purpose too, and
we colluded in that. Why stay awake? Why be alert when misery
was all around? Much better to sleep, even a drugged sleep, as
many hours as could be consumed in the long, soul-threatening
day.

Surviving the boarding home was a great struggle, but it
taught me to stay out of the hospital. I learned a healthy distrust

of the system that had sent me and the others to such a nightmare residence, expecting that their therapeutic salvage work was
done. That kind of rigid bureaucracy showed a craziness deeper
and more pervasive than any we had ever displayed. It ensured
that life outside would be as destructive to our attempts to find
health as any misdiagnosis or flawed medication we received.

Things may get worse as welfare and disability cutbacks are
entrenched. Social housing is scarce and patients are being
discharged directly to the streets or to hostels after long hospital
stays. The "revolving door" syndrome is a predictable consequence to the hopelessness of trying to put ourselves back
together while experiencing the hunger, shame, and dread of our
misery every day, all alone and without real support.

At least now we can say these things, instead of just experiencing them in dumb misery. We can say them in places where
we are heard by policy-makers and politicians who can change
the rules and bring some measure of sanity into the system.

PART THREE

Whatever Gets You Through

7.

Substance Abuse

Although the world is full of suffering, it is full also of the overcoming of it.
      —Helen Keller

We often hear the expression that someone abuses their medication or has a drug abuse problem. For those of us who have suffered from actual abuse, either at the hands of parents or psychiatrists or pharmaceuticals, the idea that we could dish it out to pills seems ridiculous. Although informed consent is supposed to be the right of the patient—the prescribing physician must tell you what you're taking and why, as well as what the downside is—in practice we aren't entrusted with that knowledge. Knowledge and information are not seen as being in our best interests by a paternalistic medical system.

Ingesting powerful chemicals with no awareness of their potential to hurt or addict is akin to purchasing ecstasy or speed from a street dealer, and it can lead us down terrible paths. That's what happened to Julie Flatt, years after she left daycare for the world outside the walls.

. . .

About seven years ago, life was going very badly for Julie. Horrible visions of blood and violence would pop into her head. When she drove, she constantly felt panic that she'd hit someone. She'd see blood on the walls that she knew couldn't be there. She'd see a heavy object and feel it hurled at someone. She developed a terrible fear of knives and wouldn't go near one.

She'd heard about obsessive compulsive disorder (OCD), and the symptoms sounded familiar to hers. So, trying to take control of things, she asked her psychiatrist to refer her to someone who worked in that area. Julie had been on benzodiazepines most of her life: Valium, Xanax, and Atavin, along with antidepressants. Her new counsellor, who specialized in OCD, told Julie that she would not take her on as a client until she went to detox to rid herself of all the tranquillizers to which she was addicted. The therapist said the medications themselves could cause some of Julie's depression and anxiety.

Julie had only gone off her meds twice before, and they were terrible times. She felt blackmailed into going off them again. But if she didn't, she wouldn't get the treatment she felt she needed. Although her family thought she was abusing the pills, she'd only ever followed doctors orders; she religiously followed their directions of how much and how often.

As fearful as ever of being locked up, she nonetheless agreed to enter a seven-week addiction program, after twelve days of detox. It was horrible. Freed from the restraint of all her medications, her OCD was "right out there." She was sure she was being punished, for no crime at all. Only two of the thirty people in the program were there for prescription drugs, the rest were in for abusing alcohol or cocaine.

"But the people were great when they weren't puking."

She went through more stress and more obsessions. They got worse and worse, and she felt she was never going to get out of there. Her throat was closing down. But she did get through the detox and was deemed ready to enter the seven-week program, paying $5000 of her own money for the privilege.

This time, there were a hundred patients, only three of whom were in for prescription drugs. The first few nights she had panic attacks that "kept the nurses up." She was given a physical and seen by doctors, who decided she should have a minimum of 25 to 50 milligrams of Anaphrinal. Thirty-six hours after the drugs entered her system, her thoughts calmed down, and she could look around.

Her days were very structured. Between 9 a.m. and 3:30 p.m. she'd go to classes where they'd tell her about the nature of addictions and the physical effect of them on the body. Though the staff would allow that addiction is an illness, they would then proceed "to tell you practical stuff that a mental hospital never does."

One hour, three times a week, was reserved for group therapy, and another hour a week was for one-on-one with a therapist. They had to attend twenty-one meetings of either AA (Alcoholics Anonymous) or NA (Narcotics Anonymous), and they were expected to do chores and to do them well. Three infractions (for example, for not attending group therapy or your quota of AA/NA meetings) and you'd be bounced from the program.

Julie had a lot of trouble with NA.

"You're supposed to say you're an addict, that it's your responsibility. But I only took what they told me to take, when they told me to take it. I felt it was the prescribing doctors who should be getting the education I was receiving. Yes, I took the pills, but they gave them to me. They have eight years of education in this mental health stuff. I'm going to them for help, and they're giving me addictive substances. Why did they keep prescribing these drugs? Why didn't they know?"

She never went back to the woman who, she felt, had forced her into the program. She found another counsellor, and she hasn't taken any tranquillizers since graduating from that program.

"It wasn't that hard once I knew I could do without them, but it meant I didn't have that extra thing to dull the pain. I recognize that all I want is for things to dull that pain, calm those feelings, but I know I can't anesthetize myself. Booze, drugs—I can't go there."

Sadly, she's also come to see her dreams of marriage and children as lost and in the same light—as simply seeking yet another way to avoid pain, another way to escape her all-consuming reality.

What happened to Julie is what happens to many women who go to doctors with feelings of anxiety that creep around the edges of their lives. The system's response hasn't changed much since grab bags of Valium were the answer. No real effort is made to understand the underlying causes of the anxiety. It's much easier to pacify the symptoms and move on to the next patient. It's much easier for the patients too, who quickly learn that some pills are nicer than others. Pills can bring on sleep and relaxation, and even make life enjoyable—until we realize we need them, physically really need them, to get up, to go to work, to get through the night.

And it's not an answer tailored just for women anymore. Pharmaceutical sales are through the roof. Men, children—eventually we may all be hooked on some form of Soma distributed by white-coated dealers. And everything will be just fine.

* * *

Barry D'Costa found himself drinking more than was reasonable after he left the hospital, so he went into an addictions program. He heard them saying things that "should have been said to me in hospital. Control was what the addictions counsellors were trying to impart—control with proper self-care and responsibility towards oneself and others, as well as being able to recognize and respond to early warning signs before everything comes crashing down."

His fellow patients were doctors and nurses and other professionals. The team that treated them was the best of the best. He found the health classes as good as anything offered in university, and the leisure and recreation group was much better than the "group outings" that had been the hallmark of the psychiatric ward.

In the groups they talked about finding a balance, that focusing on work to the exclusion of everything else was ultimately self-defeating; that leisure and recreation are necessities, not options; and that there must be an equal investment in personal, family, and work time. Barry learned that "birth family" issues are more insidious than many people recognize, and that most problems are in place long before drinking and drugs take over.

"I knew for me that I had gone through a period of excess and abuse, but never considered being an addict my prime identity. I still went to ninety AA meetings in ninety days, and I appreciated the structure and the discipline, but couldn't see myself attending 'the church of AA.' I wanted to take what I learned at the program and apply it to the mental health issues that were plaguing me. When they talked about sobriety, I heard emotional sobriety."

Every morning, they were awakened at 6:30 a.m. to do a mile-and-a-half walk through the woods before breakfast. A pulse check showed they were reducing their resting heart rate. The exercise increased their feelings of control and their ability to withstand stress. Barry took what he'd learned there and used it to enhance the fledgling self-help group he joined in Kitchener-Waterloo.

The addictions programs described here provide a practical, hands-on approach to regaining personal control. Unfortunately, they are not widely available to the poor or to those who can afford just a few days in grim, squat detoxes. Barry had insurance through the university he was attending. Julie used her savings. As you'll see, Dan got into an American program just days before OHIP stopped funding out-of-country stays.

*   *   *

Living with pain is debilitating. It is natural to seek relief wherever it can be found, and far too many psychiatric patients find ways to ease the pain that add to rather than erase their problems. For Dan Carter, though, his eighteen years as a drunk were coming to an end. By June of 1991, he was drinking forty-eight bottles of beer and one bottle of Scotch a day. In the past few weeks, he'd added cocaine to his liquids. Things were close to the point of implosion. He weighed barely 111 pounds, the flesh simply hanging on his six-foot frame.

"I was bankrupt in every aspect of my life."

He was suffering from paranoia and anxiety. His problems were no longer just physical; he was deteriorating mentally as well. His sister had had it with him. His parents were older when they adopted him, and his sister had bridged the generation gap, becoming a second mother to him. He vividly remembers the day she "slapped him upside the head" and told him he had two choices: "Sober up or die. Just do one of them well."

He was moved to take a look at himself in the mirror, and for the first time in a long time he really saw what he looked like.

Until then, he'd thought he was fine, that he looked great. Now there were no delusions obscuring what he saw. He was terrified.

He started phoning addiction treatment centres, and he found one that was holding an orientation session for family members and potential customers that same afternoon.

Dan couldn't be too far from his booze. He'd start to shake and have difficulty holding himself together. He put on his raincoat, stuffed the pockets with full bottles, and took himself off to the meeting. It was hard to pay attention, but he heard one thing very clearly. There was a three-month waiting list. He stood up, started pulling the bottles from his pockets, one after the other, and choked out: "I don't have three months."

There was nothing they could do to cut the waiting time. Understanding that he was finally serious about getting care, his sister called a friend in California who tracked down a "lock-down treatment program" that would take him immediately.

By the time he was buckled into his seat on the plane, he was starting to crash. He hadn't taken a drink since hearing he had been accepted, and now he was sweating, anxious, and fearful. A flight attendant innocently suggested he have a drink to calm himself, but he was determined to white-knuckle it. A nurse-liaison had been sent to accompany the handful of Canadians on their journey to California, and she held his hand all the way to LA.

Anaheim, California, seemed to be "a very long" city, and the drive from the airport took an eternity. Even a fifteen-minute drive would have felt like fifteen hours in Dan's rapidly deteriorating condition. He was ready to collapse by the time he made it to the sixth floor of the Martin Luther King Hospital. They put him in a glass-walled ICU, gave him an injection to calm the withdrawal symptoms, did blood and urine tests, put him on a heart monitor, and connected him with an intravenous drip. The room seemed so cold. If he'd had twenty blankets he still would not have felt warm. He weakly joked with one of the nurses: "I know I'm from Canada, but Christ, it's cold." With some sympathy, she told him the room was actually quite warm.

This was the first time in eighteen years that he had committed to making a real change in his life—in another country and in this strange city where he knew no one. Filled with paranoia, he didn't know what the next fifteen minutes would hold.

"Suicide would have been a lot less painful."

It was ten days before he could take real stock of his surroundings and eat his first breakfast in decades. He admitted to himself that although part of him was still scared to death, another part deep in his soul was exhilarated and believed that he would get a second chance.

Dan found both group and one-on-one therapy helpful.

"You could talk out all the garbage of your past in a place where everyone had done shitty things. You spend years in this destructive cycle. People won't accept you because of what you are, what you've become, so you drink more, lie more, cheat more; here there was unconditional acceptance—you built up trust and it never came back and bit you in the ass. It was a tremendous relief."

But the therapy went beyond that. As part of his healing process, he was expected to make amends with the people he had damaged and whose trust he had abused. He had to take responsibility for the things he'd done in the past, rather than wallow in guilt and shame: perfect excuses to drown himself again.

He remembers a "really nice guy" from Hamilton who had flown out with him on the same plane. One day the FBI showed up at the hospital and charged him with murdering his wife. Later, the man sent a letter to the group from his prison cell, having gone back to Canada to face the charges. He said he had no memory of stabbing the wife he loved in a drunken rage, but he knew he would have to take responsibility for his actions.

Dan spent eight weeks in the lock-down program, and then six more months attending the hospital and group every day. The hospital had outpatient lodging, a kind of highly programmed halfway house, where he stayed for four months. He was then offered a guesthouse by an engineer who'd been on the ward with him.

"I knew I wasn't strong enough to deal with the issues I had to deal with. It took me a good year before I even attempted it."

So it was a year before he flew back home to handle the mess he'd made of his life, his relationships, and his family. Some friendships could not be repaired. Some he had to break off because of their negative influence—he left behind his old drinking and drugging buddies. His parents and his sister were skeptical of his sobriety; it took them a good five years before they believed in him again.

After two years, seven of the twenty-six patients he'd lived with on the ward were dead either from suicide or accidental overdoses; only nine were still sober. Dan was proud to be one of the nine. More tragedy and challenge lay ahead for him, but he knew how much he wanted to live—as a responsible and giving adult, someone his family could be proud of.

The best addiction programs encourage personal responsibility, growth, and community, and give practical, everyday advice to the participants. Most mental health treatment programs do not do this. They don't teach that we can control our illnesses. But we can. We can learn to recognize symptoms and triggers and to respond to the "illnesses" when they re-emerge, rather than take medication that calls for surrender and compliance.

Too often, mental health patients are discouraged from questioning doctors about the diagnoses or medications. Surrounded by experts, they are often treated as children, as if everyone else knows what's best for them and they needn't worry their little heads about it anymore.

What if mental hospitals encouraged patients to go for long walks first thing in the morning, even before the medication lineup? What if they encouraged patients to learn from one another and to take responsibility for their actions as adults? What if groups learned how to get a personal handle on this thing called mental illness? What if patients spent more time outside than in, exploring the world around them? A treatment like this might give mental health patients a fighting chance to have a real life waiting for them when they are discharged.

8.

Self-Harm

You could see the wound or the burn. You could bind it,
stitch it, watch it heal.
                    —Laurie Hall

Addictions don't have to be only to substances. We can become
addicted to behaviours. Behaviours can obviate the need for
speech and can dramatically reveal the turmoil inside us.
Sometimes, they help us cope, at least for a little while, when
nothing else can. Behaviours can punish; behaviours can confuse;
behaviours can make us feel alive when life itself has been stolen
from us by medications that leave us flat and dull.

   If prisons are the best places to hone new criminal skills,
psychiatric wards and hospitals are "centres of excellence" in the
instruction of how to be the craziest you can be. The teaching is
not conscious or deliberate. It occurs through a kind of osmosis
in the closed environment, where vulnerability, fragility, despair,

and acting out get attention: the rewards are more medication to show how serious the pain is; observation twenty-four hours a day; four-point restraints; and long stays in bubble rooms with only a mattress for company.

For some, the first episode of self-abuse is so terribly frightening that they dread any repetition. Compliance, surrender, and acceptance are the only rational responses to the horror of self-abuse for these people. Their lives will be forever constricted by the psychiatric version of "chemotherapy" they receive, as debilitating as the real thing with the intended effects and side effects condemning them to a drugged half-life.

For those who are non-compliant, who are questioning, or who are still angry, the road ahead is rocky and much more dangerous. They do not see this solution as any solution at all because they suspect the experts are not all-knowing and all-seeing. These patients are viewed as resisting treatment and refusing their roles. They are labelled difficult and uncooperative. They annoy staff who become aggravated with them and leave them alone much of the time (staff on one ward I was on used to draw straws to see who would have to be my nurse for the shift). These patients strike back the only way they can: against themselves, against their bodies. This seems better than asking for a different kind of help than is offered, by staff who have already judged and interpreted them.

A case in point is the disturbing, almost ritualistic behaviour known as cutting, or self-harm. I saw it for the first time when I was on a psychiatric ward in Montreal: a teenage girl kept slashing at her wrist and arms so much that, to discourage her, the staff made her sew up her own cuts. There was nothing particularly inviting about her behaviour or the staff's reaction to it, which seemed quite heartless and cruel to the rest of us. Yet, years later, I was doing the same thing, cutting at myself, even as I wondered why.

"It's surprising how many of us took it up all at once," says Laurie Hall. She had never seen anyone do it, never heard anything about it, until her first "episode."

Laurie was on constant, twenty-four-hour observation; it was her second admission, the first having lasted only days before she'd signed herself out.

"The 'constant' was a nurse who was always knitting at the end of the bed, following me to the bathroom, making me leave the door open when I bathed or showered or peed. I wasn't allowed matches or lighters. I had to ask for a light, which I did. So I was smoking, and I very deliberately put the glowing end right against the back of my hand and ground it right in. The best part was that my expression didn't change at all. I found it quite easy to control the pain. Then I made sure she saw it. They went all mental on me, tied me to the bed."

But there were benefits.

"You could see the wound or the burn. You could bind it, stitch it, watch it heal."

It seemed to relieve the dreadful pressure of the moment, like an escape valve. Although professionals first thought these cuts were incompetent and laughable attempts at suicide, for many of us, they are actually an attempt to stay alive.

*   *   *

Pat Fowler has been part of the survivor movement for about five years—they've been five years of growth and self-learning. She was in a couple of leadership training groups I conducted through the Ontario Council of Alternative Businesses (OCAB), and she showed herself to be competent, courageous, and funny. She has deep scars that she hides under long sleeves, even on warm days. Pat tells her story.

"My mother was very dominant, and my father was passive in the face of it. We spent a lot of time being afraid because of the way she would withdraw emotionally, even if you spilled your milk. We always gave her migraines. My sister was worse; she gave her heart attacks. My brother, of course, was perfect. I was the middle child, and already the sick one, since I'd already been in hospital when I was six years old because I was so short. I remember her 'mad back'—how she'd stand rigid at the sink while my father drank. We learned to watch for that, and to be warned by it. She was a clean freak. We weren't allowed to do anything because we'd wreck it. I couldn't iron, do my own laundry, not even boil water for soup."

In her early teens, Pat developed a need to clean her hands with scouring powder that would leave them red and raw. Her mother would just laugh, "Oh look, Patty's at it again."

"I think she felt everyone was better than her, and everyone's kids were better than her kids, so we were constantly torn down."

Pat, a bright, brave, self-deprecating woman, started slashing soon after her discharge from an eating-disorder day program.

She was in her early thirties and worked as a provincial government payroll clerk when she was first diagnosed as bulimic.

"I wasn't a prototype. I had real problems vomiting, so what I would do was exercise madly, walking two, three hours at a time, really fast."

And it worked. She was dramatically losing weight, even with her bingeing. Her doctor referred her to a hospital day program, and Pat took three months' leave from work to participate. She wasn't as thin as some of the others, and she certainly was not as bad as the patients who had been admitted to the inpatient ward in critical danger. Pat became friendly with some of the people there, especially one wealthy, very beautiful woman whose father sat on the hospital board.

"I remember one day she showed up with a big scrape on her hand. I asked her about it, and she told me she'd been trying to hang a picture and cut herself on the nail. I didn't think much about it at the time, but it seemed she was always having little accidents."

Aside from work, Pat led a lonely life. She had little to look forward to except the vacations she spent most of the year planning—trips to Tahiti, Greece, and Switzerland.

Her sister believes that if Pat had not gotten caught up in the therapeutic system, all the destructive behaviours she adopted would not have occurred. Pat thinks she may be right. Being the object of professional concern and the centre of attention was like an opiate, and Pat was quickly becoming addicted to the notice she got. After her discharge from the program, she began to overdose on the pills they gave her. They had also just given her Ipicac in emergency to induce vomiting. She declares with a small laugh that she would have been a much more successful bulimic earlier if she had known there was such a drug, helping her to eat, purge, eat, purge.

As with any addiction, escalation was inevitable, and one evening she found herself playing with a disposable razor. (The trick with disposables is to dismantle them to free the blade, but she hadn't learned that yet.)

"At first it was just little scratches. I'm right-handed so I worked on my left arm. Then I bought some real razor blades. I'd be really scared before I did it, though it wasn't very, very painful. Afterwards I'd be almost euphoric."

She'd start slowly, just pressing the blade against the flesh of her arm, and then she would quickly slash. The pain was minimal. They finally admitted her to a self-harm unit, where she stayed for a month and soon adopted all the behaviours she saw around her.

"I always slashed for attention. It had to be severe enough, deep enough to require stitching. I would keep at it until I had a good one, where I could actually see the fatty tissue. It was guesswork, and a bit dangerous. They'd warned me I could accidentally cut through tendons and lose the use of my arm. Still, I loved to see the bright, turquoise stitches, loved to touch them, feel them. I cut countless times in a four-year period, visiting every hospital emergency ward in the downtown area. I think, after a while, the staff really hated seeing me come back through the doors."

The stitches didn't hurt either. The doctors would use a local anesthetic before sewing her up, except for one "son-of-a-bitch" who used staples without freezing her arm first.

A diminutive woman, Pat was 4' 8" and haunted by childhood images of herself that she despised. In her teenage years, she had piled on the weight. Her anger at her appearance fuelled her cutting: "It was . . . I'm such a freak, freak, freak, cut, cut, cut."

"I remember being tormented in grade one. I was a fat, chubby midget of a kid, and I had to wear one of those old, clunky hearing aids connected to a big silver box that dropped on my chest. As if that wasn't bad enough, I also needed really thick glasses."

She was still heavy in her twenties, which is when she began her frenetic walking and strict dieting.

"This is going to sound really pathetic, really embarrassing, but I'll tell you what I think was going on in those years I spent slashing. I hated the room I was living in. I was desperately unhappy and very lonely. I had no friends; I was still a virgin in my thirties; I was such a freak that I thought I was going to die a virgin. I didn't know back then that you didn't have to be anyone special to have sex. Mental health workers, especially male psychiatrists, were substitutes for that—for friends and lovers, for any caring relationships."

For a few years, she stayed in a nurses' residence dorm connected to the hospital where she was receiving treatment. When she was able to get her own apartment once again, it was wonderful and liberating.

"To have my own space, my own bathroom, my privacy!"

Pat had been able to find a temporary job during RRSP season. She had worked 420 hours, but in order to collect UIC, she needed something approaching 450 hours. When she was forced to apply for welfare, she was told that her refuge was too expensive for the housing costs that she was allowed and she'd have to move.

"It was like they were telling me I had to be homeless to get welfare."

She came home one day to find an eviction notice on her door.

"I couldn't survive on the street. I knew that."

She had heard about OCAB and that they were looking for a receptionist. She felt fragile and trembled through most of the interview. They almost didn't hire her, though there was no question about her ability. Once she had the job, there were unexplained absences for a couple of days at a time. She'd call in at four in the morning (when she knew there would be no one to take the call) and leave a message about feeling ill. In fact, Pat had no money for transit and lived very far from the office. She was embarrassed and humiliated by this, and didn't want to tell them. Once that was sorted out, she bloomed.

"OCAB changed my life. It was the first time I was not seen as a person who wrecks everything, but as someone with abilities, someone people could believe in. Therapists had told me I was too fragile to keep my own apartment, my own separate space. They had suggested I give up my job and my place, and move into a Sally Ann residence. That lasted all of a week, after which they sent me to another supportive housing place, and it was awful. Here I was used to living on my own, and they put me in a bed two feet away from a senile old lady who kept stealing from me."

Since then, she has conquered her shyness by standing up in front of groups and talking about her life and experiences. She has co-starred in the documentary *Working Like Crazy*, a film about survivor businesses, and she was part of a road show to England, Scotland, and Ireland that encouraged groups of survivors and professionals to push the idea that everyone can work. Recently, Pat and my sister Diana made a presentation on the same theme at a conference in Amsterdam.

Pat Fowler is clear about the effect of finding community and of working with survivors at the OCAB. She began to learn from them and what she learned was more positive than what she'd picked up from inpatients in the hospital. She was making friends and getting feedback about herself that was at odds with the "freak" she once felt herself to be. She began to tell herself not to put medical staff on a pedestal, that the people in emergency were not stitching her up because they liked and cared about her, but that it was just their job.

Though she has slipped once or twice since, the cuts have not been deep or serious enough to require stitches. She has made the decision to "never ever go to hospital ever again."

Pat has had laser surgery on her eyes so she no longer requires the thick glasses that once made her a target for the jibes of children; she has a discreetly hidden hearing aid; and she has a few lovers under her belt. She takes Paxil, an antidepressant that has helped her, and she has taken on increased responsibility at the OCAB so that she feels fulfilled and tired enough at the end of the day to sleep well through the night. She is still occasionally derailed when her old habits of tearing herself down surface, but her self-awareness and her coping skills are getting better, and she is getting used to being praised.

Diana says of Pat: "She's pure gold. I'd be lost without her. She sets such a high standard; she's such a wonderful role model for others."

*   *   *

Lee Robson was seven when she started cutting and burning herself where it would look like an accident—as if she'd been pulling the toast from the toaster or slicing vegetables—or where she could hide it. Her father was an alcoholic, and her mother was hypercritical about anything and everything Lee was and did. She was told constantly that her hair wasn't right and that she didn't dress properly. She grew up feeling worthless and insecure. She cried often and couldn't eat. Her therapist told her years later that her mother had subjected her to a kind of emotional incest, by invading her whole person, her very psyche.

When Lee was eleven, she was gang-raped by three drunken teenagers. They found Lee and her friends smoking cigarettes (being as bad as they knew how to be at that age), but Lee couldn't run away fast enough. It was brutal. And she thought they would kill her. When she regained consciousness the next day as dawn was breaking, she knew they had killed a large part of her. She went home with "body fluids dripping everywhere, with parts of my ass hanging out the back of me," and as she came in the door, her mother smacked her on the head and demanded to know how Lee could do this to her. Lee never spoke of the rape, not to her mother, not to anyone, until many hard years had passed.

She was "away" for the next six months, her mind taking her somewhere else while those around her never noticed. Her dad was in and out of jail for alcohol-related offences. Her brother was also serving time for delinquent behaviour. When she was fourteen, she slashed her wrists in the school washroom. After that, she began cutting in front of people.

One day, as she walked up the street to school, she made deep cuts on the back of her hands. They were too deep, she realized, and she got to class bleeding all over herself. The school called her mother to come and get her. Her mother was very angry, and Lee remembers her saying: "What on earth is wrong with you, you stupid girl?"

Lee later cut and overdosed, which left her in a coma for three days. She remembers waking in hospital to hear a doctor (whose first language was not English) yelling at her: "You could have been a fruit!"

Very groggy, and confused, she asked, "A what?"

"A fruit!"

"Ohhh, you mean a vegetable."

Lee was placed in a group home after it was clear that she and her mother could not live together.

"It was great for me. I didn't have to be with my mother, and I felt, at the home, that I was part of a big team. I loved it."

Lee believes she picked up her work ethic from her parents.

"You could have cops at the front door, all hell breaking loose inside, but come morning, you'd still get to work on time."

She had gone to George Brown College and taken courses that helped her get a job in the print shop of a hospital. During the day, she'd see kids sitting around outside the Ontario College of Art. Curious, she decided to prepare a portfolio of some of her more creative pieces, and she applied. She got in.

"It was wonderful, and socially fantastic. I could relate to people on a very different basis than partying or work. It really brought me out of myself. Let's face it, you don't have that same exposure working in a print shop."

She wasn't free yet of her mother's voice, which had moved into her head and was always ready to undermine, to start a downward spiral.

Lee describes it like this: "I could get home, after a great week where everything went well, and start washing dishes and drop a glass. Right away, I'd hear, accusing in my head: 'You stupid bitch, look what you did. And you did the same thing last week. And the week before you . . .' Quite soon you're mired in the devilish 'Why are you still breathing?'"

Now, rather than silencing that voice by cutting, she stops it before it enters her psyche, before it threatens everything she has accomplished. The last time Lee cut was more than a decade ago. She was in her own apartment when her mother came by and started criticizing her once again; Lee snapped. Grabbing a razor blade she slashed over and over again, the worst she'd ever done. Blood splattered the walls and floor, even the cat. Her mother "looked pretty horrified, which was good."

The hospital stitched her up and sent her back home. But Lee had learned by then that she didn't need anyone else to know how upset she was, that it was enough that she knew. And her life was starting to improve; she had more to lose than she'd ever had before. It was time to stop.

Lee has a lot of creative talent. Her home is also her workshop, and she is surrounded by cutting tools. On those days when she felt the need to cut, when anger or despair would well up, a determined Lee wouldn't allow herself to get out of bed until the urge subsided. Sometimes it would take three days before it was safe enough for her to even walk to the bathroom; she kept a bucket by her bed to pee in rather than risk getting up. Survivor Laurie Hall comments: "That desire, that compulsion to cut or burn, is the same as craving a cigarette even years after giving it up."

Lee graduated from OCA, and her great friend Diane Savard nagged her into applying to work in a supportive housing program for female psychiatric survivors. Lee worked there for one and a half years, until the ads came out about the job openings at the Gerstein Centre.

"At first it seemed absurd to me, hiring consumer/survivors to work with people in crisis. I mean, it was neat, but I didn't really get it. First, you're given a label that pretty much means you're an idiot, and then you're told that this same label can get you a good paying job." Some professionals thought that too.

Lee didn't think she had the right education or experience to make it through the interview at the Gerstein Centre, and she certainly did not have the confidence. I was part of the hiring panel. Lee still works at the Gerstein Centre, and she still learns there. She has a quiet, successful life, works full-time now in community mental health, and has learned first to be aware of and then to quiet that harsh critical voice that moved into her head at a time when she was too young to keep it out. Was Lee saying to her mother: This is how you make me crazy, or This is how I survive you? It's hard to describe how it feels to be flooded with despair, anger, and grief, as if you'll drown, or explode, if you don't ease the pressure.

For some, it is a matter of life and death.

*   *   *

I was living in temporary digs beside Allan Gardens, once again in between jobs, with not a lot going on. The flat itself was in an old building, with a separate entrance to my spot on the third floor, and there was an unfinished "deck" (a tar roof that left sticky black crap on the soles of my feet) that I could access through a window. It had a kitchen I stayed out of, not trusting that I was the sole occupant of the place, not wanting to know if rodents and bugs were infesting the aged appliances or cupboards. As Toronto low-rents go, it wasn't terrible. The neighbourhood was bleak, with the park just a place for the homeless to bed down, for crack dealers to sell their wares, and for hookers to sell their bodies. It had an entirely different feel than Parkdale. It had as much despair and poverty, but less of the streetwise toughness, less of the drug-and-alcohol-fuelled violence.

At the time, I was having an intense affair with a woman who was recently separated from her husband. (My first lesbian encounter had happened in college in the late sixties, when experimentation was the norm. More than that, it was demanded if we were to live up to the lifestyle of a downtown hippie clique. She was a boyfriend's girlfriend, blond and strikingly beautiful in the distinct Montreal mode, and we giggled our way through the lovemaking, a sweet, funny, unforgettable introduction to sex with the same sex.)

Though it didn't "take" that first time, I think my attraction to straight women stems from that experience, and not just because they were straight, but because I preferred it if they were involved in heterosexual affairs or marriages, guaranteeing it would be a brief interlude in their lives and mine. It felt safer, though I still don't know why. When I worked at Parc, we would spend a lot of social time with staff from the hospital down the road, partying at their houses deep into the night. Relationships developed naturally—I must have dated a half-dozen nurses over my time there, only one of whom was gay.

It was mid-December. Icy cold, dark, the wind howled through the park where people were trying to stay alive. I didn't like it here.

Didn't like stepping over bodies in the morning, didn't like the shouts and screams tattooing the night. Didn't like being scared.

Didn't like being left behind.

"I have to go back home for a few weeks. Over Christmas and New Year's. The children are all coming. I have to be there."

She'd known for a while, but hadn't wanted to upset me. (Any woman who has ever been the mistress of a married man knows the routine, the excuses, and the absences at those times that matter most. Being the mistress of a married woman was very much the same, but still hard for all that.) When she was around, life was better and I breathed easier.

When she dressed and left me to pack, crying, I was in an absolute panic.

I can't do this, I thought. The weeks ahead, getting through all those days, all those nights, I just can't do it.

For seven years I'd been totally immersed at Parc. It had occupied every waking moment and probably troubled my dreams. The inactivity I experienced for months after I left—finally admitting to burnout—was threatening my sense of self, my right to take up space on the planet, my justification for continuing to breathe in and out. I was already simply holding on, waiting out the dead time, holding off the depression that kept threatening—like the winter itself—to devour me whole.

It was not a good time to feel rejected or abandoned or bereft, if there ever is such a time.

In my college days, we used to heat up knives to facilitate the smoking of hashish.

I braved the kitchen, not turning on the light, and grabbed a breadknife off the counter, gingerly turning one of the burners on high, resting the blade across it, standing and staring as the red glow got brighter, and the blade started to blacken. I took it back to the bedroom (the only room I used), and sat on the still warm and crumpled blankets atop the mattress. The knife was a magic wand that would return my strength and resolve to me, the only price asked being pain. To the music of the wind and the cries of the lost, I held the blade against the flesh of my upper arm (where it would be hidden, a shameful thing, a secret thing) again and again and again . . . until the deeper, untouchable, ungovernable pain receded.

I think I slept for a time, and woke to the sound of a key turning in the lock, the door being pulled open, and light footsteps on the narrow staircase. She was the only one besides me to have a key. I grabbed my long-sleeved shirt off the floor, and did it up with trembling, clumsy fingers. She came into the darkened bedroom carrying with her the starkness of the reality of her presence, the reality of the world out there, where people did not do such things.

"I'm on my way, but I couldn't leave without seeing you again. I love you. I'll call you as often as I can. It won't be so long, you'll see."

She'd brought gifts—things that would make me laugh, make me remember, parts of her life, the one not shared with me—a music box, a pair of crystal dice, figurines. Bringing me close, she kissed me and we started to make love. Ashamed and suddenly fearful, I was fixated on keeping my new scars my secret. Impatient with the clothing, oblivious of my efforts to distract her, she pulled off the shirt and gasped, and then leaned over to turn on the light.

It was at that moment I swore off—only to myself—this dependence on self-harm to get through. The blunt reality of the angry red burns, the strangeness of them in the light, the effect on her, which of course was to blame herself, made me determined not to do this again. I would not hurt anyone I loved like this again. I swore it and meant it, and kept the vow.

•   •   •

Survivors make the same bad decisions that unlabelled people do, again and again. Sometimes it's who they choose for friends; sometimes it's how they handle their finances, if they have any to handle. It has less to do with being crazy than with being human, flawed, and recreating the past in the present. But there are some behaviours—such as slashing—that are found only within those people who've been subjects of care, of professional interventions.

People with little else in their lives can become addicted to going in and out of crisis. It's a way to hold on to those scant moments of attention. Health care workers fall into the trap of only responding to those who are in trouble, the squeaky wheels getting the grease. But the more they fix the crises, the less self-reliant the patients become. The intervention reinforces incapacity, rather than capability. Patients lose any incentive to manage their lives, to learn to handle day-to-day stress, and to handle conflict in constructive ways. A gradual institutionalization of adults out in the community is the end result.

I've worked with groups of survivors around this issue for OCAB and other agencies to get them to step back and see how long periods of time spent in hospitals, agencies, and drop-ins can inadvertently discourage personal growth, responsibility, and self-control. Real work—having something to lose—is an incentive for people to break out of that cycle, to build their lives on firm footings—not just from crisis to crisis—and to take pleasure in their own very human development.

PART FOUR

Elements of Rebuilding

9.

Straight Talk

A man cannot be comfortable without his own approval.
—Mark Twain, "What Is Man?" (1906)

After all the crazy behaviours and the psychiatric interventions have played themselves out, there is just you, and your pain— and an abyss that gapes where your next fearful footstep could fall. Where do you begin to rebuild?

"A home, a job, a friend" is a good slogan and a good start, especially for those trapped without purpose and without expectation, in dead-end, crowded rooms. Some of the survivors in this book have shown how transformative these elements can be. They are what we now require, demand even, from the mental health system. They are the minimum that we should have and that workers should help us achieve.

But what else do we need, then, to find a level of peace in the world? How can someone who's been through so much find a safe place to make a stand, a place to start rebuilding the self, from the inside out? Where do people find the strength and the simple optimism to go on?

There are things we must do, steps we must take, by ourselves.

Every individual is different, in spite of similar backgrounds and diagnoses, in terms of potential, character, insight, interests, and abilities. These differences may be obscured by labels and behaviours, by poverty and homelessness, but they are there. And they need to be expressed in order for us to find out what makes us special, what makes us unique. The failure to see us as people, not as pathologies, continues to wear us down. It is extraordinary, a kind of miracle, that in spite of having no outside validation of our basic common humanity and all that that entails, some of us cling to a sense of self that is quite different from that persona in the files that follow us from place to place. It is mostly a recitation of behaviours that sets us apart and that marks us as difficult, as chronic.

The world isn't a place that metes out fairness. There are tragedies and horror stories almost anywhere you care to look. Death, disease, abductions, famine, abused women, abused children, loss, so much of it abounds that asking Why me? is a kind of arrogance. No one is guaranteed safe passage through life, and this should tell us it's less about the suffering and challenges than what we do in the face of them.

If we allow ourselves to become embittered, riddled with self-pity, or emptied of everything but fury, we lose. Plain and simple. If we stop living, by letting fear and caution define our days, by only taking the careful, shuffling steps of an invalid, we also lose by allowing the label to become a death sentence.

We have to take responsibility for the lives we've been given. We cannot leave it to others to define us, to control us, and to limit us—not to our psychiatrists, our parents, our partners, or our siblings, not to anyone who is not us. Our lives are our own. Here are some concrete steps survivors can take to beat back the effects of labelling, isolation, and shame.

First of all, seek information.

Once you've gotten over the shock of that first episode and the trauma of that first diagnosis, you need to get to work to establish control. The first step, after things have calmed down, is to get a second opinion. Initial diagnoses are often wrong. Don't allow yourself to be silenced by the "experts." Go in with prepared questions: Why have you settled on this diagnosis? What are the symptoms you see?

Most of us have a great deal of trouble telling others what's really going on in our heads. Sometimes we may feel embarrassed or ashamed or simply distrustful, so doctors may make assumptions based on our silence or on the behaviours they see. Since the mental illness label may well follow you for life, at least it should be reasonably accurate.

Learning how to recognize symptomology can help you stave off or shorten another episode and it can teach you what to watch for in your day-to-day life. If you have worries (as most of us do) about confidentiality and about keeping your thoughts and fears private and away from parents and others, be very clear about that right from the outset. Ask how detailed your file is, and who sees it.

Be aware that your first experience of medication, especially if you were admitted to a ward, may well have been over the top in terms of dosage and effects. This is a terrible way to be introduced to pharmaceuticals, and it can lead you to believe that a chemical straitjacket is all that is available for you. We all respond differently to medication. A clear explanation of the intended and unintended effects of the pills you take will help you monitor your own reactions. If the psychiatrist brushes off questions about medications (some think if they answer truthfully their patients will stop taking the drugs), you can change doctors, ask your pharmacist, or go to the library and look up the answers in the *Compendium of Pharmaceuticals (CPS)*. Aim for the least possible dosage, or drug vacations, in partnership with your psychiatrist, if possible. If he or she balks, you may find that a general practitioner will be more ready to help. Never go off your medications cold turkey, unless you're looking for a hospital stay.

Remember you are not a disease. You have a personality, a character that will play a large role in how you cope with this illness. A general prognosis, however, does not take that into account.

Your psychiatrist is not just a psychiatrist. He or she is simply another human being, with some specialized knowledge that is filtered through his or her own life experience, prejudices, likes, and dislikes. Don't be passive in the face of his or her pronouncements. Be fully engaged, question, and learn—don't give in to the label. If you can afford other avenues of assistance such as therapists or herbal remedies, explore them, cautiously and with eyes wide open. Unfortunately, not everyone has access to costly alternatives.

It's rare in the mental health community to experience just one admission to hospital. You need to understand that repeat admissions are less about your illness than about your need to come to terms with the illness and to understand what you're looking for. Too many of us are lost when our behaviours escalate and when our desperate search for a cure lands us again and again in emergency wards and bubble rooms. We want to be fixed and to be made better. If we live long enough, we do eventually understand that we're the only ones who can improve our lives and strengthen ourselves. It can seem like an overwhelming realization—even brutally unfair, but there it is. The sooner we accept that, the safer we'll be.

And there are other experiences, side effects of being labelled, that are equally unjust. Many find themselves deserted by friends they've had for years. You need to know that this reaction is not unique to mental health patients. Divorced women, people who live with cancer, AIDS, or Alzheimer's, those who've just lost their jobs—anyone struck by tragedy learns how quickly important people fall away from them, abandon them. They also learn to value greatly those who don't disappear, as well as the new friends they make, often individuals who share the same experience.

We also may try to drive people away. One way we do this is by punishing those closest to us, especially parents, by engaging in wars of attrition—wars that usually come down to one side saying, "Take your pills, for God's sake, at least you'll be safe;" the other side blindly striking out with the only control left: refusal. This conflict is a very temporary, futile, and possibly dangerous distraction; it can keep us busy and raging, and it can delay, sometimes to the point of no return, our coming to terms with our adulthood, with our lives. You can lose the sense of time passing in these wars and it can be very hard to find your way back, perhaps—if you wait too long—impossible. You can allow your world to shrink to the boundaries of your own anger, your own sense of grievance. And blame it on the illness. Cold comfort, indeed.

Life is about growing, striving, learning, and fulfilling whatever potential you were born with. The real sickness lies in forgoing all that.

If the first thing you need is information, the second is perspective.

How many people are content with their lives? How satisfying are the sacrifices they make for their families, the deadening jobs that eat up their souls, and the increasingly faint echoes of what might have been? How many men use their midlife crisis to shift directions, to make one last grab at a less-empty existence, usually with someone twenty years younger? Not many people get to be rock stars or artists; even fewer get to lead the lives they thought they would in early fantasies of what should be. Mental illness has little to do with all the little failures that plague them, all the might-have-beens that all people feel at one time or another.

My life has been much more than it should have been. I've done more, accomplished more, than I ever expected, or that was ever expected of me. So have most of the people I've written about. Mental illness has opened doors for us, not closed them, given us purpose, resolve, and courage. It's given us challenging, meaningful, and interesting lives.

And a chance to make a real difference.

It is not helpful to believe that the universe has singled you out for destruction. Reading about the challenges other people have faced and overcome, whether it be political oppression, illness, poverty, or early abuse, will change your perspective: there's a cornucopia of stories of suffering and triumph out there. Watch the nightly news. Volunteer at a food bank or a retirement home. Spend time at an Out of the Cold program. Get out of the narrow space of your own skull.

Perspective helps you develop empathy, a much better emotion than self-pity.

Perspective can also help you deal effectively with stigma; it helps you to understand that stigma was not something tailored solely for mental illness. People will always shy away from what they don't understand, and people being people, they may not understand a lot about the many different challenges that others face. You may have been a contributor to stigma yourself, before your label was ironed on. And you may still be a contributor, if you allow shame to limit and confine you.

Develop self-awareness.

Even if you find you can't be totally truthful and forthcoming with your professional helpers, don't hide the truth from yourself. Understanding what motivates you, scares you, and leads you into self-destructive acts, won't instantly—if ever—lead you to the path of normality, but it may help you get a handle on why you seem to do incomprehensible things.

Are you stewing in anger that this has happened to you?

Are you looking for rescue?

Are you looking to make others suffer as you suffer?

Wilful blindness is only another trap. For instance, you can know and understand everything about an illness such as manic depression, including what brings on mania, and—like a junkie with a needle, like an alcoholic with a bottle—you can still be seduced by the high, by the intoxicating surge of emotions and feelings of power. And damn the long-term consequences, until you're a pile of ash inside. Swept up, you are swept back into hospital, until the next time.

Our illness is within our control, however much we may deny that it is, and we have to choose to exercise that control, rather than have controls applied externally once we've played ourselves out.

It doesn't have to be a choice between feeling and not feeling, although it may be seen as such by those who need an excuse for this addiction. It is very sad and frustrating to meet self-styled artists who believe their diagnosis is simply an outgrowth of their creativity, rather than a barrier to it. They feel persecuted by frequent admissions to hospital, often against their stated will, but refuse any personal responsibility for behaviours that guarantee those admissions: running down city streets naked; spending their life savings; accosting strangers with their formulas for world peace. And it's a given that after each episode, more medications will be prescribed, leading to more deadening of emotions, to non-compliance and a continuation of the cycle.

I used to think that I could only write well if I was depressed, tortured, and suffering. But depression, like mania, has its own agenda, and creative output is not on it.

Get involved.

Try not to live in full retreat from life.

People hang on better through rough times if they feel they have something to lose. If your days and nights are empty, psychosis can look pretty inviting. So can hospitals and professional attention. The drama involved in being actively mentally ill at least shows us that we're alive and that someone out there has to care for us when there is nothing and no one else to assure us of our value.

Any way of engaging with life that is positive and life affirming, any way of focusing attention outside the narrow framework of self, can immeasurably improve your chances of staying "sane." You may not want to reach out; you may feel that you shouldn't have to settle for less than others get out of life. But you will never know just what you're capable of achieving, even with this gorilla on your back, if you never try.

Going back to school, finding fulfilling work, hobbies, or volunteer activity, sharing whatever talents you may have, finding groups or new friends who are also looking to get back to life, finding workers who encourage rather than discourage your efforts to rebuild—all this is infinitely more effective than simply existing parallel to life.

Yes, it's hard, and yes, it's scary. So is being isolated and bored. But with every successful step you make towards becoming a full person, the stronger your resolve becomes to stay on that path. Setbacks become just that, temporary setbacks on the road to recovering the self.

Seek out role models. There are many more than ever before in the long and terrible history of mental illness.

Be cautious about self-medicating.

Many more of us self-medicate than admit to it. It can be quite wonderful, for a short time, to find a drug or bottle that helps us to relax, to feel human—until we develop a dependency and an addiction that compounds our problems.

Be aware of the risks associated with these different escapes, if you're determined to try them out. Stick to the least-harm principle that is now coming into its own in addictions treatment—meeting some of the addiction's needs in order to moderate it.

When you're especially fragile, drugs like crack, acid, coke, or ecstasy can spin you into psychosis, and make it difficult for you to find your way back. Some people can't seem to tolerate even the milder drugs, such as pot, without going off their rockers. For others, the softer drugs help them get through bad times, and it becomes a viable choice, albeit an illegal one.

The rule of thumb is: Be careful.

The most critical elements you need are courage and patience.

You need the courage to try, and try again. Recovery is not an "instant karma" experience, it's a process, one that demands that the person afflicted be an active participant.

Finding what works for you can be as frustrating as finding a medication you can live with, if you feel you need and want that medication. But when you find where you fit, where you're useful and productive, it's a better high than anything you'll get from mania or street drugs.

You may see yourself as weak, broken, and fearful, and discount the fact that you have survived more than most people could bear. Though you feel that your courage is in short supply, it is there, dormant perhaps, but there, and you can tap into it, add to it, a little at a time.

Use your anger.

Using the anger at your core, harnessing it instead of turning it against yourself or others, goes hand in hand with courage. The anger that branded us and fuelled the behaviours that brought us into care, may ultimately be responsible for our successes. That anger refused to accept the judgments made against us. That anger caused us to question, to swim upstream, and may well have saved us from lifetimes of chemical lobotomies.

But you have to be ready.

You have to be at a point where you are weary of living from crisis to crisis; you have to be done with constantly running from or acting out the inner pain so that others can see it when you can't find the words to express it—from slashing to overdosing to setting fires; you have to understand that the help offered or imposed on you does not and cannot do what you need it to do. Even though you don't know what it is you do need.

The first step is always the most difficult, but once you've started moving, once you've resolved to take back your life, you're already halfway there.

10.

Moving Forward with a Purpose

You don't know how stupid or how smart you are till you actually try.
— Diana Capponi

It's important to get a handle on your illness as early as possible, because you'll eventually have to make up the ground lost during each episode. Either that, or you will live the life of a fifties mental patient, and that's a bleak prospect indeed.

When I was in my boarding home, I wasn't aware of time or of opportunities passing. The place shielded me against life out there—against that messy, hurried, real world where monsters lurked at every corner. As bad as the boarding house was, it was a kind of safe place. No one else there was thinking about next year, or even next week, unless cheque day was coming. We accepted our exile, and learned to make do.

We were seventy lives fading away, without ever really knowing ourselves, or our neighbours, or the city we lived in. What we needed to do, however, was to take charge of our lives, and to address the challenges that faced us. The sooner mental health patients do this, the better. There are no shortcuts; it's hard work, sometimes painful work, with few people cheering you on. But you're doing this for yourself, for your future, and you can be your own cheerleader. There are some practical ways to get started.

It might help to keep a journal of your efforts, so that you can see progress, even if others can't. Start small; don't throw yourself at life and expect it to embrace you. For instance, if you had a breakdown while attending school, you might want to start back with one or two courses, not a full load. If you haven't been able to leave your house, a walk around the block can be a major accomplishment for the first few days. Then extend that walk farther and farther until you are used to being outside and you lose the feeling of vulnerability that kept you inside.

Survivor businesses are great ways to get back into a work rhythm, but there may not be any available in your province. You might want to look at starting one up, or at finding part-time work in the mainstream. Each accomplishment will trigger a hunger for the next one.

Some of us need something other than ourselves to get us moving and to keep us moving, and that's fine: children, spirituality, community organizations, ambition, even a paycheque—all are quite legitimate motivators. It doesn't matter how you get moving, just get out and do it. And if you experience setbacks, don't waste time beating yourself up. Learn from them, and start again.

The label of mental patient will destroy your life only if you let it.

*   *   *

My sister Diana found satisfaction in rebuilding herself and a shattered community. Watching her over the years, I've been amazed at her tenacity and strength, and I've wondered where on earth they came from. She used to be so afraid of people that when she first started to work, she hid in the bathroom to eat her lunch. But she never lost herself in the "Why me's?" although she had reason enough to become bitter and hateful. She chose instead to give back to her community in spectacular ways. And in doing so, she began to understand herself; she began to grow and learn and teach.

There had been so much raw violence in our house, so much naked hate, that I never thought we would have secrets from each other, child to child, parent to child—all the ugliness and brutality seemed to be already out there. But there were secrets. The secrets were so terrible, so shameful, that they never slipped out, no matter how out of control the fighting got. Years after we'd all gotten out of the house, when my sister Terry was getting crazier and crazier, psychiatrists told her that she must have been sexually abused as a child, that she had all the symptoms. She absolutely refused to accept it.

It never happened.

But it did.

Even today it hurts to think about what kept my mother with my father. How did she see the daughters that he violated: as competitors? as willing participants? Did she really think that the couple of times she witnessed his incestuous behaviour were the only times? Did she think that he'd stop because she told him to? It wasn't until decades later that our mother admitted to Diana what he'd done to her.

"Mummy said she'd caught him 'necking with me'—her words—in his green Chevy. Remember that car? I was disgusted, I almost died: you mean he was kissing me on the mouth?"

Our mother had yelled at him, threatened him, and told him to keep his hands off the girls.

Diana never really wanted to know the truth. But there are moments she recalls—remembered feelings, remembered fears.

"When we moved from Two Mountains to Chomedey, he had to do some stuff with the old house, and he'd take me with him. I felt special, you know, how much he loved me, and I never wanted to go back home, where everything was back to the usual."

Even as an adult, she feared being alone with him, feared he'd do something, especially when he was being nice and friendly.

Diana and my brother Michael were the last two children to be trapped in the house. Grade school and high school were places of great torment for Diana, as they were for me, but for different reasons. I kept mostly to myself, before being "rescued" by teachers who found some potential in me. The younger kids were more social; they were aware of what was going on around them and how they were perceived.

"We couldn't hold our heads up in the neighbourhood, or at school. Everyone knew about the Capponis."

Diana had been pulled out of school at the end of grade nine because our father said there was no sense keeping her there since she was too stupid. He sent her out to work. She came home one day to see Michael being beaten up again.

"I told Mummy I couldn't stand it anymore. I couldn't stay for her and Michael. The next thing I knew we were at her sister's house, the three of us. It was like the Waltons—a real family scene. I remember my uncle taking me down to the basement bedroom, hugging me, and it felt like such a relief, until he stuck his tongue in my mouth."

Diana was desperate to escape—to escape family and to escape herself—and she found a way. For a while it seemed like that particular hospital bed had the Capponi name carved on it. I would be packing up my few possessions, experiencing my usual ambivalence about leaving the ward, and Diana, suffering from psychosis, would be filling in admission forms, ready to take my place.

The bed was in a four-person room that had an extra door cut in one wall—a door that swung back and forth easily. It was the first thing we saw in the morning and the last thing at night, and it led to the shock room. A couple of times a month, our room became the recovery room, as semi-conscious patients, heads lolling, drool dribbling down their chins, were walked or carried through that door from their "treatment" to our beds. It was an unspoken threat to us. We saw it as a form of capital punishment for those who failed to improve.

A nurse who'd become my friend outside of the hospital as well as in warned me that Diana was in much worse shape than I was. But that is all she'd say; I didn't know that Diana was shooting heroin and living in her own nightmare.

I was still living and working at Channan Court, a huge psychiatric boarding home, when my mother put Diana on a train for Toronto because she didn't know what else to do. Diana was in and out of psychosis, trying to stay clean for her infant daughter Julia, but full of fears, real and imagined. She was admitted to Queen Street and stayed for some months. Julia lived with me in the front office that was now my bedroom. (I thought this was better than trusting the CAS to hand the child back after Diana's stay in a psychiatric hospital.)

When Diana was deemed ready for discharge, she overheard them talking about referring her to places that sounded suspiciously like the home I was in. So she curtailed their efforts to locate another boarding home, and took a basement room in Channan Court. Better the devil you know.

Heroin is a terrible drug, a deadly drug, and it thrives in poor neighbourhoods where there is no promise and no hope that tomorrow will be better than today. Diana's bleak, damp, dark room in a place where suffering was the norm was a fragile, ineffective barrier against the lure of the drug. She had to get out.

The long, uphill journey for Diana began at a program called Focus on Change. Sole-support mothers met once a week at the local library and daycare was provided for the children while the mothers talked and compared notes. Then there was a five-days-a-week school program for mothers at Eastdale Collegiate. They provided teachers who could do assessments and help clients explore the job market—even find placements—while the children were cared for.

"It was really good to get out of the boarding home and to be in a room with 'normal' women."

Diana learned that she was eligible for student loans and that she could get extra money while still collecting welfare, effectively doubling her income. She decided, having only completed grade nine, that she wanted to go to college. The staff didn't feel it was time; they worried that she'd be setting herself up for failure, but she persisted. She applied for the course to become a corrections officer. During her time as a junkie, five years of "walking death," she had been jailed a few times for vagrancy and for possession. She was familiar with the criminal justice system. She'd had horrible experiences and had seen how women were treated; she wanted to make a difference.

"You're absolutely nothing; your voice means nothing. The female guards were more male than the males."

Young girls were left in the same holding cell with women already serving time for murder or manslaughter, who'd been brought in for more court appearances.

"There's nothing tougher than a tough broad."

Diana was part of a group interview for the corrections officer course. She submitted the papers they asked for, and couldn't believe it when she was accepted into the program.

It took a lot of determination to get herself and Julia up and dressed in the morning, to take the long bus ride to the daycare, and then set out for the long subway ride to the college. My sister Terry encouraged her: just get there, just show up, the rest will happen.

"The class was mostly kids, younger than me, just away from Mummy and Daddy; but there were others who'd roughed it out for a couple of years. I made excellent friends, and was confident enough to get annoyed at some of the things that were being taught, at some of the assumptions made about why people get themselves in trouble. As long as I could make points clearly, and back them up, the teachers were okay with being challenged. I 'came out' as a crazy during the abnormal psychology class. I remember talking about Channan Court and the people trapped there. I was gaining confidence; I thought I had every chance of changing my life."

She had a human being for a Family Benefits worker, a nice man who told her she was entitled to first and last months' rents; when she won a scholarship that first year, Diana was able to move out of the grim boarding home into the top floor of a duplex.

Terry and I went to her graduation ceremony. The young girl whose father had told her she was too stupid to be kept in school stood on the stage and beamed at the audience as she accepted her certificate.

She worked part-time at Parc that summer, and heard about an opening at Nellie's, a shelter for battered women.

"I had no intention of applying; this notion of a place run by a feminist collective scared me. Paul Quinn [the same man who'd been such a support to me] had another Parc staffer pick up the application form, and hounded me until I completed it. He even made sure it was sent in."

She was shortlisted and eventually hired.

"I remember literally skipping down Broadview the day I got my first paycheque chanting, 'I'm rich, I'm rich, I'm rich.' I even photocopied it to keep."

Nellie's was a housing program for women escaping abusive relationships. Diana saw women whose stories were very close to home. She had to face the same issues over and over again, trying this time to win, trying to salvage lives.

"It pushed all my buttons, sometimes making me so angry; all the frustrating, system barriers—almost like it was a deliberate strategy to force women to give up their children. It really helped that the staff had time apart to meet, to talk without fear with each other about feelings and anger. It helped legitimize what I was feeling, going through."

And there was guilt.

"Why had I been so fortunate? There was no real reason for it.

Here I was getting paid for working with women who were just like me, some who would make it out, some who would be defeated."

She had moved from a point where she had no sense of her own strengths to where she was slowly recognizing them. She was beginning to understand how anger can be an effective motivator, rather than something destructive turned inward on the self.

*   *   *

Our father died years ago on a Thanksgiving weekend, and his passing hit Diana very hard. It threatened everything she'd accomplished—her job at Nellie's, her home, her hard-won peace. But after his death there were things to do, to arrange, so she went into operational mode. Her feelings could be put on hold until she was home again. Terry and Diana stayed at our father's house while they sorted through his papers, and Diana was struck that this unhappy man had lived by himself in what was really a family home, a five-bedroom house outside of Montreal. Every cupboard was fully stocked; every modern convenience was there.

"At the funeral, I stood over his open coffin, and stared and stared—you know how lifelike they can make a body seem—and I had to be sure he wasn't breathing."

Terry was the oldest and lost in her own pain, her own memories. She was determined to break through the hypocrisy of the service, and to punish those who must have known. She said to anyone who came up to her before, during, and after the service: Do you know what he did to us?

"I felt guilt, that I'd hurt his feelings by refusing to see him. I know, I know, but that's how I felt. Then hugely angry, that there was no recourse now for him to be held accountable. I still don't understand why he did what he did; he didn't have to beat up defenceless kids. But it was the stuff he shouted at you, the names he called you over and over again that were almost worse than the sexual abuse, than the beatings."

Every evening our mother would call, her fury fuelled by his death. His escape from the consequences of his actions was something that she must now endure. She'd lose herself in horror stories to the point where her voice "hurt my eardrums."

Diana tried going back to work, but she herself was losing it, ambushed by feelings held at bay for so long.

"For three months I holed up in my apartment, and just ate."

Diana doesn't do therapy; she doesn't trust it. She remembers being on the subway after a session once, on the day Marc Lepine savagely massacred fourteen female engineering students in Montreal. She fantasized about having a machine gun, targeting one man after another, in her mind at least, blowing them away.

"These feelings were very extreme for me, very scary, and I put it down to the experience of therapy dredging everything up."

She couldn't let our father destroy her again. Even the thought of going back on the needle made her physically ill. She pulled herself back together and returned to work, to her friends. After eight years at Nellie's, she took up a position as executive director of Fresh Start, a survivor cleaning company that had grown out of Parc and that had run into trouble early on.

"There were twenty survivors who just wanted to work. I didn't know anything about running a business, never mind what community economic development was. It was learn-on-the-job time. And I really learned. People who I thought could never hold down a job, those least able, could get to work on time, do the job, and do it well. Real pay for real work was part of what motivated them, but there were also expectations to live up to, the importance of expectations and the belief that they could do it."

This experience led her to believe that work opportunities should be available to our wider community. A tiny group of five people submitted a proposal to the provincial Ministry of Health, and the Ontario Council of Alternative Businesses was brought to life. Under Diana's leadership, ably assisted by a board that Laurie Hall chaired, they moved from a budget of $76,000, enough for one staff member and rental space, to an annual $587,000 from the province, and a further $400,000 from the City of Toronto and the Ontario Disability Support Project. They have 11 full-time employees at the head office and 700 people currently working province-wide in OCAB-owned businesses.

"The power of showing, not just theorizing, that people can work, really impacts communities where the businesses set up."

As does the power of showing ourselves that we are so much more than what one man tried to make us believe.

*   *   *

Five of them travelled the two hours to London, Ontario, by train: Diana and her partner Brenda, Diana's daughter Julia, Pat Fowler, and Dini Dinsmore, OCAB's regional coordinator for Toronto. They were all nervous and a bit giggly, not sure what the evening held in store for them. They were going into an environment where few survivors had been invited before. Diana, nominated by Centennial College, was to be one of a handful of recipients of the Premier's Distinguished Alumni Award.

It had been totally unexpected, that first phone call from the people at the college. Recalling a very different time of her life, just at the start of her long struggle out of illness, addiction, and poverty, Diana remembered how she'd stood with an infant tucked protectively in her arms, spurring her determination to make it.

"You don't know how stupid or how smart you are till you actually try."

I remember holding my breath a lot, as she fought temptation, fatigue, and her demons. Though I was there, I could not do it for her.

The event was to take place in the huge, central ballroom—tables were set up, each with flowers and glittering wineglasses, and there was a large video screen to view short documentaries about each winner. It was all alarmingly real, and much more important than they had thought. First the little group of survivors had to attend a crowded cocktail party "filled with suits, filled with normal, prosperous people," from which they quickly retreated, carrying fancy hors d'oeuvres back to Diana's room to catch their breath and work up their courage. They weren't in Kansas anymore.

"Holy shit, it's like the Academy Awards!" Diana thought to herself, dying a little as the five sat at a table towards the front of the ballroom, after they had finally worked up the courage to take their places. Queen's "We Are the Champions" played as the first recipient went up to accept the award and give a short speech, introduced by a short video.

Diana was second up. She very much wanted to do well; the college had been good to her and she recognized her obligation to them. But she was shaking, and her voice quavered just a little as she spoke the first few words, showing her emotion and the overwhelming nature of the moment.

"It was so emotional, to see Diana almost overcome. We were so proud," Pat tells me. "It was wonderful that she was being recognized by the public in such a big way, and even better that it was finally coming from outside our own community."

Not so long before, (unsuccessful) provincial Conservative leadership candidate Jim Flaherty had proposed jailing the homeless, the majority of whom suffer from some form of mental illness—in their own best interests, of course (as if there were empty apartments just waiting for them, and work and opportunity that they stubbornly rejected in favour of hypothermia). It had galled many of us who knew full well how government inaction and massive cutbacks had contributed to thousands losing their homes and hopes.

Diana's voice got more powerful as she talked about her battle to make it, what acceptance into Centennial had meant for her, and how she'd been enabled to move out of the poverty/addiction trap. She spoke of OCAB, and introduced Brenda, Dini, Pat, and her "beautiful daughter Julia," who was now crying. In a room she suspected was filled with Conservative supporters, she leaned forward to the mike, and ended with a message to Flaherty: "And Mr. Flaherty, you can kiss my butt."

One heart-stopping moment later, the room erupted in a standing ovation.

Afterwards, Pat says, "People swarmed her. And again in the morning, even at the train station. People were congratulating us for just being associated with her."

It was an extraordinary moment for our community, a rare recognition of the struggles we face and can sometimes overcome. Most of our battles are fought out of the limelight, in solitude and silence and with an excruciating awareness of our difference.

*   *   *

Religion can be a source of much pain, guilt, and anger for psychiatric survivors. Or it can become what some may call a panacea, the "opiate of the masses" that Marx claimed. I have met both Christs and anti-Christs, a couple of prophets, and even some presumptive Satans while in mental hospitals (never a Napoleon, though). For me, however, and for Dan Carter, religion provides another kind of healing. Both of us believe that the lives we've lived, the paths we've taken, and the tragedies we've endured have a purpose behind them. Both of us use our lives, our pain, and our experiences as examples for others; both of us find this reason enough to accept the past and the present.

Dan owed his sister his life—the new and better life he was leading in his tenth year of sobriety. He'd always thought she was happy; she'd never given him reason to think otherwise. She'd just passed her fiftieth birthday, and seemed to embody success, living as she did with her husband and their fourteen-year-old adopted son in their million-dollar home. Yet, at 2 a.m. on May 17, in the year 2000, standing alone in the kitchen of her house while her husband, son, and the maid slept upstairs, she plunged a butcher knife into her chest, not once but five times, making no sound "though it must have hurt like a son-of-a-bitch." She then dragged herself up the staircase, finally collapsing in the bathroom off the master bedroom. The autopsy showed she was "stone-cold sober" at the time. The police at first suspected the husband, unable to accept that someone could kill herself in such a violent and hugely painful way. After a thorough investigation, it was ruled a suicide.

Life doesn't stop presenting challenges and new crises just because you've had quite enough, thank you very much. There is no generalized immunity, no fair and equal distribution. When his brother Michael had been killed, as terrible as that had been, Dan had thought, "This is the worse thing that can ever happen to our family." It seemed as though it would confer some sort of immunity against further tragedy. But he was not immune, and his sister's death was another heartbreak.

Dan has the same absolute awareness as I do of God acting in his life. He remembers that at his time of greatest need and readiness to reform, everything fell into place against all odds. When he needed rehab, Dan could have been turned back at the American border like the man in line ahead of him. Because of his uncontrolled drinking, Dan had a criminal record for writing a bad cheque; but he sailed through customs. Days after he was accepted into the California program, he learned that the Canadian government had just announced its intention to stop publicly funding medicare for Canadians seeking treatment in the States for drug and alcohol abuse.

"You tell me all the mojos weren't working!"

He feels God has given him all the tools to do what he has to do.

Unlike Julie Flatt, who, given the option, would rather not have been born, Dan says that even with everything he's gone through, he would not trade the life he's lived for another.

"I'm here to do a job."

As a televison host, he has a potential viewing audience of a million people; he speaks to many groups about his life and his learning; he knows people find comfort and strength through him because they come up after each speech to tell him.

He and I can't have this conversation with many others; faith makes most people almost as uncomfortable as mental illness. This faith, however, does not scatter roses across our paths or remove those agonizing times when the sense of personal failure and the inability to help those closest to us overwhelms us. It also doesn't help that sense of foreboding: What next?

Dan and I also have diverging views—he says he is terrified of death, whereas I am still impatient, but not precipitous. His sister's death has shaken him to his very foundations, but he knows that God "gives us the lessons we need, though I wish this was one lesson I could miss. You go through or over so many hurdles in life, you get so busy with crisis after crisis that finally you have to say, 'Wait a second here, I don't know what life is about anymore.' You have to take time out to rebuild and reflect."

And he's done just that, separating from his wife, and moving into his own space. He goes to a therapist, and takes just enough medication so that he doesn't snarl at the people he works with, and doesn't destroy what he's built up. He was never tempted to use his sister Maureen's death as an excuse to regress to old ways of dealing with pain. It had a lot to do with seeing how tormented his parents were.

"There is nothing worse than seeing elderly parents cry. It's just horrible, and so terribly sad. It stays in your mind."

At this point, he wants to discover what love is; he wants to experience the normal joys people feel on warm, sunny days; he wants to get back to himself. And he keeps reminding himself: "You're a participant, but you're not in charge."

●   ●   ●

My own current level of peace with God was hard-won, after I learned I was still capable of misleading myself, of attributing motivations and intentions to Him that proved false. Shortly after I started to work in Parkdale, I was hit by a cable company's van. At first I didn't know what was happening; things got fuzzy and there was this sense of a huge force pushing me, as strong as hurricane winds, but I was surrounded by silence. For me, God works a lot like that. He's a strong, irresistible force that sends you where you fear to go, for reasons of His own and that have nothing to do with the direction you've chosen or the path you'd prefer.

Laurie Hall saw the Father in the Sky as a mirror of her own dad. At times, so would I, especially when the stresses of life caught up to me, sending me down strange roads where threats seemed everywhere. Judgment and punishment in this life and the next—deserved and undeserved—seemed to be all He offered. At other times, my relationship with God would be less tormented. I would read and study to understand what purpose I had and the reasons for the pain and suffering I had witnessed for most of my life. Accustomed to taking on blame and responsibility, I would conclude that God wouldn't have had to resort to forging me by fire if I had been a better, stronger, more giving person, and therefore the fault must be mine. I would look at holy books and agonize when I'd read that God gives no one more burdens than they can bear; if that was so, then what were my hospitalizations about except my personal weaknesses and failures? I would also feel guilt for not appreciating this gift of life He gave us, for my frequent suicide attempts, and for the multitude of sins I'd committed.

Believing that God works through people, people in all walks and stages of life, I'd feel guilty that I was such a poor instrument for Him to use. Every time tragedy struck, I would feel Him at work, correcting me, directing me, and He scared me to death.

I've come to believe, in this relatively calm moment of my life, that I get into trouble when I resist the purpose I'm supposed to serve, the role I'm supposed to accomplish. When I get too comfortable (and there were not too many opportunities for that to happen) or too lazy, I'm not out there doing what I'm supposed to be doing. If this is delusional, so be it. We all have our delusions, and some are more widely shared (therefore more acceptable) than others.

I've also come to better terms with God, having spent some angry years turning my back on Him, though I was still aware, still conscious of the fact of His existence. I feel Him in my life; I always have, for better or for worse. I've learned not to focus on my shortcomings and sins so much, but rather to concentrate on doing the good that I can.

Not expecting to win heaven or avoid hell, I would choose nothingness after this life is done. I can't imagine myself so different from who and what I am as to enjoy any eternity no matter how wondrous. Fighting for good is simply a better, more worthy occupation than signing up with "the dark side," whether there's a God or not, whether there's a final accounting or not.

Allan Strong had spent some time on his own search for something larger than himself. He studied Buddhism for a while, and then Marxism. He even became a card-carrying member of the

Communist Party—they used to call their headquarters on Cecil Street in Toronto the "Church." Allan briefly became a Baha'i, before finally finding his place in the Mennonite community.

Julie, on the other hand, believes she has a reciprocal relationship with God. She prays frequently for support and courage, especially before making a speech.

"I lay everything at His feet, all my worries and fears, and then go to the podium and talk."

She shocked me when she said she'd rather not have been born. She has accomplished so much in our community of survivors. I assumed she would share the same sense of a fair trade-off that I feel. I wanted to argue with her, convince her, but that's not right, either; we are entitled to feel what we feel. And I remind myself that when I look at the children playing in the schoolyard opposite my place, I too feel the weight, the burden of the years ahead of them. A future sadness stands in stark contrast to the sounds of laughter and life bubbling up from them.

We have to keep moving forward in life, keep building the skills we need to replace old defences when things are relatively quiet and peaceful, so that when the inevitable downturn comes, we won't be set back so far. And we have to find a purpose, a reason to keep going, a reason to keep check on self-destructive acts that only serve to discourage us and those around us.

I was taught powerlessness early in my life; it was the main feature of my life, and it still plagues me in my inability to affect the lives of those closest to me, to protect those surviving family members from struggle and pain.

•   •   •

*My mother's life had been hard, even with the lifetime prescription
for Valium that had continued to be mailed from Montreal long
after she'd moved to Toronto. The drugstore that supplied it closed
just around the time of my brother Michael's death from AIDS, just
when she was most vulnerable and tormented by memories and guilt.
At the same time, her oldest daughter, Terry, who for years had been
the most settled, stable, and successful of all her children, was not
doing well. Terry's increasingly eccentric and disturbing behaviour,
fuelled by an all-consuming rage, showed clearly that the destruction
begun at our father's hand—so many years ago—was continuing to
bear poisoned fruit. My mother was angry that her husband seemed
to have escaped all this so easily, dying from a massive heart attack,
while she was left to deal with all the horror. Guilt, warranted or
not, the endless onslaught of tragedies big and small, and poverty
always just around the corner, made everything worse as she tried
to compensate for the emptiness and unhappiness she felt.*

*I'd felt so much guilt—piled on in childhood and added on ever
since—that there was literally no room to feel anything else
towards her. This in itself was guilt-inducing. Like Barry, I'd
always thought that if there had been no children, her life might
have been radically different. She might have had a life. Everyone
loves their mother, even if they don't particularly like her. Even if
they fight and yell, there is something approximating love there;
yet, I still felt nothing but pity for what my mother had gone
through, for what she was forced to face.*

I wanted her to have some measure of peace and comfort, and to find whatever happiness she could eke out of her remaining years. Though there was some contentment, there was also the awareness in all of us that there would be no end to the assaults on our lives, that Michael's hard death was just the beginning.

My mother died in her sleep. My stepfather awoke to find her cold and gone. A major heart attack stole her away under cover of night, rescuing her from life. Diana, the youngest now, went over to their co-op apartment before the coroner arrived, and reported that there was no stress or fear or pain on her face, that she had died without suffering through any of that.

It seemed the best possible end, an unexpected kindness, a gentle stealing away in the night.

Now there were just four of us left, the four daughters.

I worked out my own comforting delusion. Where it came from and why, who cared; it felt right. I was sure, absolutely certain, that I would follow my mother. That that was God's plan. This certainty had calmed me, and made me almost cheerful in my day-to-day life. After all, I had high cholesterol levels, was a relentless smoker, was over fifty, and was too used to poverty diets to take on a tofu-and-bean-sprouts lifestyle. With both parents dead of heart disease, the odds were in my favour. I was free of the suicidal thoughts that had accompanied me through most of my life: it was simply a matter of time—a matter of coasting through the months, even years, remaining. It was all downhill from now on.

I suppose that all sounds a bit odd, but because I'd lived with thoughts of death since I was ten years old, it was a profoundly comforting thought—not a frightening prospect—as long as it wasn't the result of a debilitating disease or a plane crash. For months, I made certain to tidy my room every night, so the ambulance attendants and coroner's crew wouldn't judge me too harshly. I left a large envelope on my desk with instructions for anyone finding my body—living alone requires such planning.

There was even a heady feeling of victory under layers of bone-deep weariness; I would get to the end with some legitimacy and experience a natural death that wouldn't leave an aura of failure and defeat for others to deal with. I had been detaching myself from relationships and human encumbrances since 1995, leaving people's lives and circles, reducing the ties and obligations most take as a given, all this with an almost Buddhist-like resolve. It's not just possessions that weigh us down, keep us in the game, obscuring the goal—it's also the drama of day-to-day existence—all the players who need you to participate in their lives. It's not something to try to explain to others. It just is.

Though I cared about people, relatives, and friends, I kept a stern and self-disciplined distance. I didn't want to follow all the twists and turns, to be powerless again in the face of their individual destinies.

So I spent my time waiting.

Sometimes we can move seamlessly from a form of sanity to what in retrospect seems a little crazy, without realizing we're over that diagnostic line, heading for trouble. My thoughts had moved from the rational stance of waiting out the rest of my time, to believing that any day now I would be called up. These thoughts had the weight of a real commitment, one I accepted without reservation or examination. The stress of the past few years had caught up with me.

You should never let down your guard between crises, though all survivors do. We allow ourselves to cave (just slightly), to buckle (just a bit) under the weight of what we've endured. We feel we don't have to be as strong anymore for anyone else, and the nightmares come galloping through the breach, as I found when my small world was threatened.

I thought I had a deal with God and that the rented room that was my home, my refuge, and my safety would be my last place. There'd be no more moves, no more beginnings, no more first nights in strange buildings with all the lights on, waiting. I wouldn't have to listen for the sounds of ugly, sudden violence, the skittering of rodents, watching, watching from the corners of my eyes for that first heart-stopping sight of occupying roaches. I was too old, too tired to endure all that again.

Almost as soon as the other tenants were told that this building was up for sale, people started making plans to move out. Shrugging off the inevitable, couples broke up, lives altered, rooms emptied one by one. Is that normal? I wondered, watching them go, cars stuffed with their belongings, rented vans filled with furniture. Some cried as they said goodbye, but the tears were temporary, there was an undercurrent of excitement, of expectation and adventure.

"You're going to try and stay? Good for you."

There are things you can't explain to "normal" people—why I wasn't looking for other places, why I was risking homelessness by not checking the for-rent ads in the papers. This was my home. If God was going to take me, He'd take me from here. It seemed like a bargain He'd agreed to. And broken.

I refused to move and got a legal clinic to take on my case, until a bizarre and lengthy ruling from an adjudicator went against me. Under threat of appeal, the landlord finally dropped his efforts to evict me, and put the house up for sale again. In the midst of all this, I felt vulnerable, hugely uncomfortable with the rage that had built up inside, paranoid, and betrayed by God. I was unable to trust enough to sustain important friendships that had been the mainstay in the past decade of my life. I felt that, whatever it says in the holy books, He had miscalculated and this was more than I could bear.

I remember trying to out-distance the internal waterfalls of loss and the pain, walking furiously through downtown streets, almost doubling over from the force and intensity of it, sure that I could not survive this latest assault. Trying to ignore the siren call of old habits, old solutions.

And then the other shoe dropped.

A phone call.

Terry was dead.

She'd talked herself into a temporary pass from a psychiatric ward, and when she didn't come back, the hospital notified the police. They checked her house, got no response, and left. We'll never know the cause of death, but since she was found with a television remote in her hand, it probably wasn't suicide. I don't think you'd care much what was on if you were about to kill yourself.

During a prolonged heat wave, she had collapsed, and lain dead or alive for days, her body so decomposed it became part of the floor of her house. Diana went to that tiny house, which Terry had bought with thousands of dollars in cash she'd carried around with her for weeks, and found it much like Michael's room when he was in the throws of dementia. Terry had scrawled strange things on the walls; it was chaotic and dirty; the basement was filled with brackish water.

Immediately, the world became unsafe. I was psychologically thrown back into childhood, where one twisted man controlled every aspect of our life; it seemed in a way he was back, more powerful and vengeful than he ever was while alive.

She was my big sister, and I admired her greatly. She introduced me to Bertrand Russell and other philosophers, capturing my imagination with thoughts much bigger than the limited visceral responses that were the norm when living under constant threat.

Terry was ambitious, determined, and tightly wrapped. In high school, she spent most nights studying in the unfinished basement, away from the noise and turmoil, the screams and shouts, single-mindedly pursuing the grades that would win her a better future. Back then, educated women could choose between teaching and nursing as temporary careers before marriage—for something to fall back on if your husband turned on you, or if there wasn't one to be found. Back then, too, children were told that hard work would bring success, and success was defined as a middle-class lifestyle.

The rest of us in the family had mountains of trouble at school, which we attributed—thanks to our father—to a lack of intelligence and ability, so Terry's scholarship set her apart. She was also the first to leave home, after she was accepted into the teachers' program at Macdonald College, far enough away from home that she would have to live in residence. I remember her crying as she lay in her bed across the room from me the night before she was to leave. When I asked her what was the matter, she choked: "I'm leaving home, and I can't even say goodbye to my own father."

Though I hurt for her, I couldn't understand her pain— in my mind I would have been throwing a huge party, not regretting for a moment the kind of parting—ecstatic just to be getting away. Terry never lost the longing for real parents, for parents who were the way parents were supposed to be.

The tragedy lies not so much in my sister's death at fifty-four as in her later life. Terry raged, oh how she raged, at what she'd lost or never known. It was a rage that consumed and transfigured a talented, intelligent, at times hysterically funny woman into a furious dervish whirling maniacally through the past and the present, forever looking back, and never letting go of what should have been.

For much of her adult life, Terry had taught elementary school, paid her bills, and earned her salary and the disability pension that would—when she could work no more—cushion her fall. She was married; she lived with her husband in a house they owned; they travelled a fair amount. When members of her immediate family needed financial help for education, or shelter, or food, she provided it. She overcame the social phobias of her youth, and though she didn't have many close friends, she had a few.

Quirky, yes. She was certainly tightly wrapped emotionally. Damaged early in her life by our father, nonetheless by the standards of our times she was the Successful One. But there was that emptiness, that black pit many of us carry within that is never appeased—can never be appeased.

It doesn't stop us from trying: with food, drugs, alcohol, and other self-destructive behaviours, with varying forms of therapy and hospitalization, anything and everything that could make us feel whole. And when we find all that doesn't work, either we learn to live with that pain, or it swallows us.

If later life had been gentler, if the crises that assaulted us had come further apart or not at all, she might have been able to continue to live in the artifice of her carefully constructed world to its natural end. But in our family we know that they come in waves, another and another and another, so that just keeping your footing is close to impossible. There's no time to rebuild, and barely time to breathe.

Terry knew that, and said that, while we coped with the agonizing fate of our brother Michael. She said this will be like a hurricane through all our lives, ripping us apart. Ripping her apart.

Her notion of the social contract—of hard work and diligence bringing rewards—had been challenged by her failure to have a child. She'd suffered through debilitating and crazy-making hormone treatments and artificial insemination, first demanding that we support her efforts and then furious that none of us had made her stop. She was on a disability pension and spent her days "watching the Flintstones.*"*

At times she seemed to be blanketed in layers of fog, and simply not there: disassociation, post-traumatic stress disorder, her mind was in full retreat. She said the doctors were telling her they believed she must have suffered from early sexual abuse, but she was sure they were mistaken, remembering only that "wrongness" that she'd felt when he'd stood watching his children in the bathtub.

I don't go to funerals, but I went to her memorial service—and it was good I did. Sometimes, we can mistakenly believe that madness is a twenty-four-hours-a-day, seven-days-a-week preoccupation. Certainly, the only times I'd heard from her over the last few years of her life were the long diatribes she'd leave as phone messages, three or four in a row. Then, weeks later, she'd leave another triumphant one saying that it hadn't been her who'd left those messages saying terrible things, but "someone else." I wondered if she was falling into the chasm of the "multiple personality syndrome" label. It was especially chilling that she'd use the same words my father favoured when he "disciplined" us—an evil kind of possession that showed how tormented and lost she was.

When we were still able to talk to one another, I tried to warn her of the danger of the path she was on, as did Diana. Terry felt that I had stolen her life, that I was living—through my writing and my friends—the life that should have been hers. It only exacerbated bad feelings when I tried to say that it really wasn't anything special—she would have made it special if it had been hers.

I warned her too of the corrosiveness of jealously. She replied that there was nothing bad about it, and anyway, it wasn't just

me—she was jealous of everyone. She lived almost totally in the
darkness of the past, and refused to come back into the light.

There were pictures at the memorial service, one in particular
of the five of us children posed on a beach somewhere. Diana says,
"If you didn't know, it's like looking at the Brady Bunch." She feels
the impulse to update it, to show outcomes: Michael reduced to a
bundle of sticks in a bed at Casey House; our mother white-haired
and wild-eyed lost in her own delusions; and now Terry, once a
shining light, left to rot in the heat.

Still. The room was crowded with people who worked with her
when she could work, with her family and friends. It was impor-
tant to know there had been a larger life, a fuller one than the
awful, accusing phone calls and letters would have suggested. At
one point, I started to smile, thinking she would appreciate having
gotten out before me, finally giving me cause to be jealous of her.
Her ex-husband said during his talk at the service that her death
had released her, that it was a mercy.

Three more deaths in the family, on the heels of my father's:
mother, brother, and sister. In spite of their youth, they were all
seen as deliverance rather than tragedy. That says a lot.

*   •   •   •*

After Terry's death, I did not cut myself; I did not overdose; I did
not walk into emergency and ask to see a psychiatrist; I did not
make midnight calls. I held on. Though I felt the ceiling collapsing on my head, I held on.

I played music; I talked to God; I walked miles; I remembered my obligation to my community and the work I still had to do. Everything I had built up in the past few decades—every connection, every individual, every accomplishment, every strength, including my spiritual beliefs—came into play and kept me going instead of yielding, instead of giving in to the horror, the grief, and the fear.

There is no point in life when we are guaranteed that nothing more will happen to us, or to those closest to us, and that we will sail atop calm waters straight on to Valhalla. We must use every opportunity to strengthen and challenge ourselves. We must weave ourselves a safety net from the fabric of relationships, from our external connections to the world. We must have reasons to push on, to push through those times that terrorize us, and make it safely through to the other side.

Here I am, calmly working at my desk, still in my room, writing these words, a year since Terry's death. It's been more than two years since my mother's death, and though there is so much sadness at the core of me, it does not destroy, it teaches.

11.

Accepting Difference

Hey Pat, I've been going through a bit of a hard time over the past couple of weeks, struggling (mainly) with issues surrounding close relationships, and feeling angry with having depression . . . angry at depression, I suppose. So, to get to the point, I have a couple of questions . . .

1. How can I turn to friends for support (with depression) and not have them scared off or think that I am fragile?

2. How can I rebuild the relationships I've lost because of depression?

. . . I want to show my roommates that I am a competent and intelligent person and not small and pathetic. I feel really small and pathetic most of the time, around most people. Perhaps I need to conquer this insecurity before I expect others not to see me that way. I want to show my friends that I have come a long way, and have become a stronger person since my "descent into darkness."

The journey for wellness will continue, some days rockier than others.
                    —e-mail from Cheryl Gray

There used to be men and women who came into restaurants and cafés and solicited money by handing out cards that identified them as deaf-mutes and that had the sign-language alphabet on the back. Whether or not it was a scam, I found the concept interesting: this is my disability; this is how to speak to me. I would love to have such a card; it's such a clean, clear way of explaining difference and how to get beyond it. I suspect, however, that my card would be too dense, too crowded with small type, footnotes, and riders, to be of any real use:

> "Hello, I am a psychiatric survivor trying to get by in the world, trying to strengthen myself, and require that those who wish to be my friends recognize that I am a work-in-progress, that I need time and space to rebuild, and that my reconstruction efforts may be derailed by the negative judgments of others. If you wish to be my friend, it is important that you respect these efforts, not undermine them, that you engage with me on the basis of all that I am and want to become—including but not limited to the pain that lies at the heart of me, no matter the guise in which it presents itself.

Dependence and need are traps for me, and for you. Please don't encourage either. But be gentle in your speech and manner, for wounds have left me raw and bleeding and without defences, whether or not this vulnerability is obvious to you.

I have been made different, and that difference must be kept in mind, for me to be safe; I am also the same in much of what I am, in much of what I want, and that too must be kept constantly in sight. I crave equality in relationships: friends not therapists, lovers not keepers. If that's too much to expect, then walk away. It will save us both a lot of grief."

Sometimes it seems as though there is no middle ground for psychiatric survivors. Either we're seen as weak and helpless, or, when we become politicized, strong and scary. Projecting a strong image is not easy for a mental health survivor; it can't be turned on and off, and after a time the need to do it can feel more like being trapped in a prison than a fortress. Everyone wants to be understood, of course, but to gain that understanding mental health patients must reveal more than feels safe to them. Like Cheryl, we learn that our strangeness, our otherness, can be used as a weapon against us. Trust becomes a complicated minefield pocked with suspicion, doubt, and hurt. I came to the conclusion that it was better to hold back, to accept that challenging the perceptions of others is a losing game; it's much better not to play. Such is the individual nature of our expressions of pain, and equally individual choices and methods of dealing with that pain, taught by experience; we learn by the lives we've led and the relationships we've shared along the way. This chapter suggests some strategies for facing the illness together.

One of the important ways to develop self-knowledge is through the daily interactions we have with others. Through our more intimate relations, we can learn even more about our wants and needs, and our ability to love and be loved. We have to be ready to build these relationships and we have to choose them very carefully. Mentors are fine, but we need to avoid Svengalis who are operating out of their own needs to transform and reshape. And we have to guard against repeating bad patterns, bad choices. My sister Diana, for example, has learned to be wary of those to whom she immediately feels a strong sexual attraction; she has learned to turn away from temptations rather than allow her past to repeat itself.

It is critically important that we have a strong enough sense of ourselves to withstand the casual assaults on who we are and to find people who will encourage that strength and awareness in positive ways. We have to be ready to be a full partner with someone who also wants a full partner, rather than sending out or responding to "change me, save me" vibrations that undermine that equality.

As well, we have to have a strong sense of our own worth and entitlement, and this can be tricky when we don't feel we're worth much. You may find, because you're the one with the label, that you constantly second-guess yourself: Should I be angry at my partner? Do I have the right to question his/her activities? Is it just my sickness that makes me suspicious of his/her behaviours? We need to judge people on their actions, however unpleasant that may seem; it is the clearest indicator of intentions and truths.

If you say to your partner, it really hurts when you say or do such and such, and he/she continues to say or do it—there's a problem with your partner, not with you. And it's a problem you must ensure your partner then deals with, if it's not to become your problem. Staying with someone who doesn't respect the sensitivities you've told him/her about, who seems to use them to hurt or attack, is a losing game.

Phrases like "you're too thin-skinned" or "you're too oversensitive" are calculated to shift responsibility away from the person doing the damage to the person receiving it. It is a truism that you can feel more alone in a relationship that isn't working than you've ever felt on your own. On the other hand, it can be quite intoxicating to be in a mutually supportive pairing, where each person is striving to grow and learn.

It is a hopeful trend that, given the opportunity and the desire, psychiatric survivors are finding satisfying relationships. It is another sign of our efforts to build our community and that we are finding our own ways to live successfully in tandem with our partners.

*   *   *

Part of growing beyond the cycle of illness and rejection is being able to understand the impact your illness can have on others, from their perspective, and to engage in their response to it. As mental health patients, it is harder than it sounds to see and feel, even to care, about anyone else's distress when your pain makes you incapable of empathy. I am reminded of a survivor who said to me: "I was talking to my sister the other night. I told her I was smoking crack. She turned around and called my mother, and now my mother is bugging me, interfering in my life. I'm mad at both of them. I wish they'd just leave me alone."

We can't have it both ways. There is often a clash between our impulses for independence and dependence: "Leave me alone, but come save me." It's a no-win situation for the parents who bear the brunt of a child's frustration and anger, and who just want their child safe and cared for. It's also no-win for the child "patient," who is overcome by feelings of confusion, failure, and loss, and who strikes out at those closest, at those within reach. Talking to good, caring parents who are in the midst of these battles is always heart-wrenching; they are overwhelmed by their child's behaviour as he or she rages against the label of mental illness. It seems to be the pathology, the sickness itself, that is at work in their child, rather than an angry response to being labelled and set apart. But the child has not become the disease.

In responding to the disease, however, parents (and even sometimes the afflicted individual) can overinvest in the specific diagnosis because they are relieved to have an explanation for all the strange and scary behaviour. They certainly overinvest in the prescribed treatment, which is usually medication of one sort or another. It seems clear-cut: a mental illness needs a pill or injection to control it. Why won't the "patient" accept it?

Though friends, family, and mental health workers are often filled with simple relief that the big and obvious suffering, the strange and frightening psychosis, is controlled and alleviated, as patients we are left in the wake of the illness with our alienation, frustrations, and even fury. No medications can touch these emotions.

We are left to ourselves.

In facing the disease together, there cannot be equality if one partner sees him- or herself as caregiver and the other feels constantly watched for signs and symptoms. Normal mood swings become suspect and worrisome; we can feel at times as if we're seen as more like a disease on the verge of an outbreak than a person capable of the full range of human emotions. Parents and partners should not become dispensing pharmacists who ask, "Are you taking your medications?" This question can become a great irritant and the ground for constant battles—a test of understanding, obligation, and personality over pathology.

There is, therefore, a great obligation on the diagnosed individual in a committed relationship to communicate, to keep real, to be responsible, even at those times when all this seems impossible. And there is an obligation for the parent or partner not to typecast their loved one—not to see everything as disease-related.

As you work together, it is helpful to view the mental health system with the same wary skepticism required when approaching a used car dealership. Parents need to conspire with their child to get the most out of the system, to understand the limits and side effects of the medications, to comprehend the often elusive nature of an accurate diagnosis, and to recognize the importance of finding a doctor who is able to establish an empathetic and informative relationship with the client. All the learning and degrees in the world can't make up for a cold, indifferent demeanour. Ideally, we should be looking for a warm, empathetic individual first, one who has the added credentials of expertise in the field.

As Kathleen Mock wrote: "Ineffective communication often reduces the accuracy of a clinician's diagnosis. Indeed, research shows that clinicians allow the patient only eighteen seconds to present the story of their illness before interrupting. Additionally, the same research shows only two percent of those patients ever get the opportunity to complete their story" ("Effective Clinician-Patient Communication," *Physician's News Digest,* February 2001). A few minutes with a patient in an emergency ward cannot give the doctor a clear sense of the person, of the triggers, and of his or her response to pain and distress. No one, especially no one who is fearful and freaked out, is going to be totally forthcoming to a stranger who appears to be judging them.

Nor is a child likely to tell the parents everything he feels or fears. As much as parents want to know what's going on in the doctor's office during closed-door sessions, the right to confidentiality is precious to survivors. If we can't trust the doctor to keep secrets, then we won't tell any.

Children can feel the same hypersensitivity coming from parents as they do sitting across the desk from the "healers"—the vigilant watch for clues, for evidence of disappointment, frustration, and rejection. If parents sit down with the child once the first episode subsides into some version of calm and enlist the child as an ally and an equal in the effort to beat back the worst aspects of mental illness, both will regain some sense of personal control. Parents should not act as if the child must now accept invalid status; they must keep reasonable expectations front and centre. Do some research together, but keep in mind that most material is written from the perspective of the medical model, and therefore has limitations. Take from it what is useful, and leave the rest behind.

Too often, survivors try to fill the black hole of inner emptiness with shovelsful of raw grievances in an effort to feel better. We paralyze and corrode ourselves with the "could-have-beens." It can be enough to preoccupy the rest of our lives if we allow it to. We are not the only individuals on the face of the earth who've suffered challenges, who've been dealt nasty hands, though sometimes it's tempting to forget that. Remembering who you were and what you wanted before your diagnosis should be a place to get back to, not a place from which you're permanently barred.

Ultimately, we are each responsible for how we live our lives, and what we do with the time allotted to us, illness notwithstanding. Understandably, our parents, siblings, and friends may want to keep us safe, protected from the pressures and stresses of life. A small part of each of us may want that too, but we will not find contentment in a half-life, sheltered from the world.

Though some, such as Julie Flatt, may believe that they can never have what everyone in the world is supposed to want, such as marriage and children, many have indeed been able to find partners to enhance and support their lives. Some survivors hook up with others who've shared the same experiences, but others build on relationships with "normal" men and women. They are creating real lives and real homes for themselves. They are having and raising children if they choose. They are going out to real work, paying taxes, building retirement funds, and—most importantly—they are giving back to their communities.

None of this happens overnight, and it can't come about while we are still drowning in need—or when we're still so raw and hypersensitive that trust is held hostage to perception. We may believe that "being normal" is not an option for us; we know we don't react the way others do to events and crises, to words and expectations. As I have said, we have to define our own version of what's normal for ourselves, and those who love us have to give us the room to do that.

Conformity of thought and behaviour is the greatest good— we learn that very young. Not fitting in at home or at school, not fitting in with a treatment regime, not fitting in anywhere is viewed as a threatening, antisocial crime, and intervention is the punishment. The real crime being committed daily, however, is society's failure to be a tolerant community, to allow those who are different to express that difference in a safe and productive way.

It's hard to come to terms with difference; it always feels like loss. Labels are self-fulfilling; this is something we've known for decades. They make the child feel anger and shame and to hate that part of him that doesn't fit, that excludes him and makes him a target. There is no celebration of his difference, unless it includes high academic success, musical talent, or something exceptional. (Like soldiers, mental health patients try to pick up the pieces of the lives they led before they went off to war, before they saw things, did things, felt things, that permanently altered how they see other people, how they see themselves. Refugees, torture victims, concentration camp survivors: often there is no road back to normality.)

As survivors we have to create a normality tailored to us. In order to do that, it's important to talk with others who've been in the same places and shared the same fears. It can be terrible to find yourself constantly judged and found lacking by those for whom the world is a safe, reasonable, and accepting place by people who contribute to the fabric of society in traditional ways: with 9-to-5 jobs, children, cars, homeownership, and credit cards. As survivors we can exchange coping strategies; we can talk about the hurtful assumptions people make about us, and how they add to the weight of our lives. We can come to see that our survival is in our hands, and that we have a right to make choices that help us to get through, even when those choices aren't understood or well tolerated by others.

It is very freeing and very liberating to find that, in the context of our early lives, the way we live, the things we require to keep us going, make perfect sense. When Julie Flatt tells me about the mornings she wakes up and something's missing, something that enabled her to get out of bed and face the day, something that was there yesterday and will probably be there tomorrow, I know those mornings as I know myself. No amount of censure from those who love you, no persistent nagging or characterization of your need to stay in bed with the covers over your head as laziness or giving in, helps. We know what we need.

This can open us up to criticism and to accusations of selfishness or misinterpretations of motives; part of maturing, of finding a safe place for oneself, is to accept that we may not be understood by friends and family or mental health workers.

But there are other times when the fact of our difference can strike us like a club.

·   ·   ·

In 1984, Laurie Hall thought that she'd found "shelter from the storm" when she was given a bed in supportive housing; a mainstream church group ran the house for female psychiatric patients between the ages of sixteen and twenty-one.

"The house was very fifties, with dark wallpaper, mismatched furniture, and everyone walking around in skirts. I was told at the initial interview that we were expected to attend the church of their choice at least every second weekend, pray before meals, wear skirts when in the house, and refer to the female staff as Miss or Mrs. So-and-So. There were no Ms's. Their curfew wasn't terrible, 10 p.m. on weeknights, midnight on Friday and Saturday. They asked a lot about my psychiatric history. I had a couple of charges for arson by then, and I was told that if there were any suspicious fires during my tenancy, I would be asked to leave. I wanted to ask if there were any other arsonists in the house, since it didn't seem fair, but I thought better of it.

"By then, I'd been living on the streets for a year. I thought, this will be good for me. In my mind, I was in survivor mode. There was a bed with clean sheets, food, a hot meal for supper and stuff to make lunches. I'd been smoking dope pretty heavily every day, so I thought it'll be good that I can't do that here."

Laurie had gone back to school to take a special veterinarian assistant program, which she was determined to complete. Having a safe place to stay made it that much easier.

The house had five full-time staff to cover twenty-four hours a day, seven days a week. They had worked together a long time and "were super, super Christian and all quite lovely. They lived out what they believed, the basic tenets of every major religion: treat people how you'd like to be treated; don't judge unless you're in a state of perfection. They were never preachy and you knew you'd be accepted whatever you said or did. I watched how they treated us, and how they treated each other. You know what it's like, the first time you see genuine respect and kindness, the first time you learn that it's not all violence and power and death."

When she'd lived at home, she'd been dragged to Sunday School by her mother, but as soon as she was old enough, Laurie stopped going.

"I'd thought about God a lot. He was someone who always knew what I was up to, the Great Big Judge in the Sky. It was so patriarchal, the Father. My father was so abusive, and it seemed like they put the Fathers together, in my mind, anyway."

She didn't like the church the staff made her attend. It was evangelical with lots of dancing and singing and no liturgy to speak of: "I liked the guitars and the flute playing—that was beautiful. But on the whole it was more like a dance party than a church service. The priest's sermons were shit, all happy happy joy joy."

Still, seeing the staff living their faith got Laurie asking questions about their beliefs. It sparked her interest in reading the Bible for the first time, especially the "bottom-of-the-pit Psalms," which she liked the best.

She was especially fond of one woman who worked there, Miss Jones. Laurie found her easy to talk to and non-judgmental, which was very important to her. Then Laurie fell in love with one of her classmates. It was her first affair, and she was extraordinarily thrilled and happy. Needing to share this momentous news with someone, she chose the staff member she trusted the most, expecting Miss Jones to share her excitement.

"All I'd ever seen from the staff was acceptance and support, but she sat there stone-faced. It seemed I'd crossed a line big time."

Laurie's first love was another woman.

Miss Jones told her, in sombre tones, that she'd have to tell the rest of the staff about this development.

"Although I knew being gay was a social no-no, I hadn't thought about the religious angle."

They gave her Bible verses to read, verses that quite explicitly railed against homosexuality. She had to endure many "psychologically based" talks with the staff, where they told her that women who've been treated badly have difficulty attaching to men, but that she shouldn't give up.

"It was a mind fuck, and it took a long time for me to sort that out."

Already uncertain about herself, this publicly funded supportive housing program could have spelled an end for Laurie. [Which is why, when George W. Bush talks about faith-based initiatives, I get chills up and down my spine.] Having workers tell you that God hates you is especially despicable.

Miss Jones was the child of missionaries, remarkably naïve, and lacking any street sense. After Laurie left the home, she began sleeping with her former worker.

"It was wonderful and horrible."

After each tender episode of lovemaking, Miss Jones was riddled with guilt and fear, she'd swear she'd never do it again.

Laurie went with Miss Jones to her church, a different church than the one the group home had forced her to attend. It was Anglican, but the priest was very, very right wing. "It took me years to figure out that he was also very antigay. The thing was, though he was incredibly homophobic, he was also very intelligent and subtle, weaving his poison into long, entertaining stories. I'd have been gone the first day if he'd stood up and said exactly what he believed."

But it got even more intense, when she was offered an "exorcism" to help with her anger, or so she was told.

"There was a big group of church people, most of whom I quite liked, who met during the week to pray and lay-on-hands. I was already the mental one in the church community, so I wasn't too surprised when they asked me to come meet with them. I think I was even happy for the attention, and I went. The first thing that happened was that the priest took me into his office and said he had something that the bishop made them get signed by anyone who underwent the procedure. Just a formality, he said, but it was a disclaimer so I couldn't turn around and sue them, I guess.

"After that, they had me sit in a recliner chair, while all the people in the group gathered round, each of them taking up positions so that everyone could lay at least one hand on me. Mostly the one guy, the priest, would talk, and the others would join in. They started with a guided meditation, just a calming thing that I was quite happy to go along with, since by this time I was scared shitless, sitting there with my eyes closed, wondering what was going to happen. I don't remember a lot, don't want to, but they were trying to toss out the bad spirits of my anger (saying 'Begone!'), and they slipped in a 'banishing of the spirit of homosexuality.' It lasted about an hour, and then we all sat around and drank tea."

Miss Jones finally ended her affair with Laurie, saying she just could not do this anymore, that she was risking eternal damnation. Laurie must have felt like a despoiler, a sexual anti-Christ out to corrupt the souls of the innocent. Laurie reconciled with God in spite of all the human interference she'd encountered. That reconciliation started when she heard about a gay church, MCC.

"I thought, given everything I'd been told about gays and God, how could that be? It took me about a month before I could get up the heart to go. They say at that church that you can always spot the first-timers. They're the ones sitting crying in the pews. . . . MCC has the same basic tenants as other churches, but they add: do you think that a God Who says the things He does in the Bible would say gays and lesbians are horrible? . . . And I said to myself, of course, of course, why has nobody in authority ever said that to me before?"

It's a wonderful moment, when you realize that you're worth loving.

And it's not just sexuality that can set us apart, that can set pathology's radar glowing, identifying difference as disease, as my own early experience with psychiatric wards showed. Not accepting the externally defined path for your life, knowing it's simply not for you, is not a sickness: self-actualization, the search for purpose and identity rarely is.

*   *   *

There are times when we're supposed to set aside our personal feelings, which are based on experience, and join with families and the mainstream to celebrate holidays that are designated as "joyous." To refuse to be a part of them is viewed as pathological and leads to more guilt and pressures to conform. We have a right and an obligation to do what is necessary to survive, and that must be respected.

December 25, 2001

My least favourite time of year, a dislike and a dread shared by many psychiatric survivors, is Christmas. There is, to my mind, a reason it comes cloaked in the misery of cold and wind and grey days, dead trees and dead grass and dead icy fingers clutching for the heart. All over the airwaves, inescapable on radio or television, ersatz people celebrate ersatz joy. Public mourning, public joy: it's all the same to me, and something to be avoided at all costs.

There's such a long lead-in to the day—weeks and weeks of anticipating the worst, dreading its actuality and the pain it will bring—that it's almost a relief to have it arrive, because then at least the end is in sight.

I do my best to mitigate the damage that will be done, the way one does with any looming disaster, as though I lived in a trailer camp and the siren has sounded early warning of an approaching tornado. I go to ground.

Some years it is easier than others to do what's necessary—to stock up on supplies of cigarettes, books, pop, food, coffee, and treats. Every year, like Y2K preparation, I get ready to self-isolate, to carve away the rest of the world, and to reduce my boundaries to the four walls of my room while the season howls unrestrained in the hearts and minds of those less fortunate, those out there naked in the emotional maelstrom. For me, it's a kind of choice. There are places I could go, and people who would welcome me, but doing that would be even harder than this aloneness. There would be prolonged expectations of social intercourse and continuity that I could never live up to.

"Name your poison," as the bartender says. I've named mine.

It shouldn't be surprising how many of us over the years have found this day excruciating, resonating as it does with the ideal: family and friends and giving and getting. The tyranny of the majority in full force, and the failure to feel the same way is viewed as unpatriotic, unnatural. Yet again.

There is always the obligatory piece in the news on Christmas dinners for the homeless and the poor, shots of old men and tired women looking thankful, plates piled high—the cameras never follow them back to the streets, to the heating grates and abandoned cars and semi-sheltered doorways that complete the night. There's nothing "feel good" about that, and we must protect the sensibilities of the season, project the warmth of good and generous feelings and the sense that no one is left out, left without. Our sense of the world we live in is as mythical, as artificial, as Santa Claus and Tiny Tim.

I worry about people worrying about me and go to some lengths to reassure them about how I will deal with the day, although explaining myself is a hateful and often futile exercise I mostly refuse to do. I worry about hurting people with my absence from their lives, but a little less now that my mother is gone. I know how easy it is to personalize, to create and swallow blame, when it's not *about blame or anger or anything except getting through. Getting through, whatever gets you through, is our mantra; to come out the other side reasonably intact, reasonably unscathed can be enough of a miracle for the times.*

For the past two Christmases, I was incredibly cushioned. Last year I was asked to mind a house and a dog for friends who were spending a month in Vietnam: it was at a place filled with freezers of food; with a dog I adored who adored me too; with music that could be jacked up to muffle any internal, insidious voices; with trust, responsibility, and wads (it seemed to me) of cash. Surrounded by clear evidence of well-being, even love, the day passed almost without notice faraway from this room and its window carved out of ice, from the wind and snow and cold inside and out. And that makes the anticipation of this year even more dreadful.

Still, this year the snow has not fallen. The weather is manageable, the heat working to counteract the drafts blowing through the cracks, and tonight I will go with a friend—who is equally disenchanted with the season—to see Lord of the Rings. *The hype about the movie began during one of those times when I was preoccupied with thoughts of death, though, unusually, it was death by natural causes I was thinking of. It occurred to me with some surprise that I would like to live long enough to see it. It was pretty much a novelty to me, putting riders on a death wish.*

It would be abnormal in the extreme for me to "joyously" embrace the season. Looking back over the decades, through the hell of childhood and adolescence, through the beatings and shout-

ing and screaming and blue-black bruises: all days were there to be endured, gotten through, all nights bitter since they led inevitably to mornings. Each morning I woke up to the same house, in the same bed, in the same torturous captivity, where anything bad could and often did happen, and during the holidays there was so much more time to devise grand and little horrors, with the backdrop of Christmas carols and talk of Jesus' birth.

Better to have those hours of relative safety when he was at work or we were at school, when fear could be set aside until the car engine growled to a stop in the driveway: Daddy's home.

Since then?

I've had Christmases on hospital wards, in boarding homes, in rooming houses, mostly bleak and fraught with the pain of others that I could not diminish. The exceptions were when I was working at the drop-in—Parc—where I didn't have to remain passive and powerless through the onslaught of the season, where I could make, with just a little effort, a little difference. I would spend all night Christmas Eve alone in the cavernous former bowling alley, with rented Monty Python and Marx Brothers movies, stuffing and cooking four or five large turkeys for the meal on the 25th, fending off skittering mice and the roaches that did death dances while trapped in the glassed-in, stovetop space for temperature, timers, and clocks.

Other exceptions were those early years when my niece Julia was young. Getting to my sister's place early in the morning, stomping around and slamming the door to announce to the sleepy kid that Santa had just left the building, I felt her real wonder and joy as she approached the tree with its mountain of brightly wrapped packages. There was a kind of victory then, smiles and laughter and hugs that are much more a child's right than fear and pain.

Still, with the passage of time, with the wearing down of the spirit, it's gotten harder to shake the stark memories of my early years, the sounds and brutal reality of those times, the encompassing awareness of the thousands of children still trapped in poverty and abuse, self-blame, and difference. While the radio relentlessly plays "Joy to the World" and "I Saw Mummy Kissing Santa Claus," I retreat into myself and my thoughts, into simply enduring as well as I can what must be endured. Not through the destructiveness of self-pity, but through the compelling need of self-preservation. Unlike the Grinch, however, I do not begrudge any real happiness that people find in this time. It is reassuring that some families like coming together, some parents are able to find room in their hearts for their children's welfare and well-being, that an ideal is still kept alive in substance more than form. It is a triumph, especially in our rapidly disintegrating world.

No doubt there are psychiatric terms for this focus on the pain of others, for the state of the world, certainly more terms than have been created for the ability not to see and really feel, which is loosely labelled normality by the majority. But those of us who know can't deny—shouldn't be forced to deny—what our experience has taught us. Not that we're asking for "Songs to Beat Your Kids By" to be given equal time with "Little Drummer Boy;" we just want the acknowledgment that there is a terrible consequence being carried by those least able to bear it—a seasonal consequence of want and despair. It is strangely liberating to know that in our own community we share a larger truth, a greater awareness of all that Christmas is and isn't, and by our numbers confirm that madness isn't ours alone. The demand that we all share a Hallmark vision of the season that has no place in our hearts and minds is a cruel absurdity.

I find it telling that, as members of our psychiatric survivor community come into positions of employment and responsibility, they make a concentrated effort to reach back and create safe spaces for people to be on this day of all days. They open their businesses for parties, meals, and commiseration, thereby recognizing and remembering and—more importantly—doing for others.

•   •   •

Difference does not equate with disease. Our experience and our difference are what define us. The greatest gift any relative or friend can give is to accept that difference and the way it plays itself out. Giving people options, such as I've been given at Christmas—"If you'd like to come, you're welcome. You don't need to call, just come"—gives us room to breathe and takes away the guilt that erodes our confidence and our sense of self.

For every bad patch, for every reminder of loss and flare-up of pain, there are days of accomplishment, days of laughter and loving; we need to remember that, to get us through. Very few people walk unwounded through life, and fewer still manage to avoid unintentionally wounding others. It takes us back to self-knowledge that provides the means of relief: knowing what helps, what hurts, and the courage to do what is necessary to ease our way.

Even when others can find no sense in it.

Julie said it best: "I don't want to feel like I'm less than I am." Those words strike a chord in all of us who've felt we don't measure up, that we're a disappointment, that motives are attributed to us that have no validity. We are people who live with chronic pain, and sometimes, just sometimes, it can overwhelm us. But we'll be back tomorrow.

Bigger and better than before.

Conclusion

Today, lines of chairs are set up inside the mall at the Queen Street site of the Centre for Addiction and Mental Health, a sprawling complex of buildings in Toronto's west end. The chairs break into the stark greyness of the cement mall and face a podium and long table at which a ceremony is slated to take place. It is such an insignificant moment in the greater scheme of things, yet it looms large for those of us with enough history to detect seed change at this institution—the Out of This World Café (OTW) is changing hands. The mall is a vast place of cement with a scattering of tables around the edges, as though people fear the centre—too much visibility and echoing vulnerability. The centre has always pushed us out and back against the walls. It may be one of the coldest places on earth, yet it's supposed to be the heart of this "caring" institution.

The OTW was a vocational rehabilitation program at the Centre that offered a coffee service for inpatients. Now it is being divested to the Ontario Council of Alternative Businesses, moving from a kind of sheltered, therapeutic endeavour to a survivor-run, survivor-controlled business within the walls. The Out of this World Café, reborn after eighteen months of negotiation, is the first of its kind in the province and probably in the country. There will be a bigger, more formal ceremony in a few weeks, but everyone involved wanted to mark this day, the actual day, when the papers are signed by representatives from the hospital and from OCAB.

Even without the identification cards hanging around their necks—like so much primitive juju warding off similarities and symptoms—the staff of the institution are easy to tell apart from the clients. Good health in their faces, good clothes on their backs, and confidence in their steps—they contrast remarkably with those huddled uncomfortably beside the metal stacking chairs, people who have been rendered almost immobile in the winding cloth of poverty and madness. That contrast is how it's always been; it's the institutional way of things. But today there's a breath of difference in this airless place.

Here and there in the small crowd, however, are some who have torn off their bindings and who stand as tall as any staff member, their presence challenging the norm. They wear their craziness, even their relative poverty, with panache and pride, as a part—only a part—of who they are and who they constantly struggle to be. Our whole survivor history, the past and present and the possibilities of our movement, is contained right here and held within this moment of time.

There is the traditional madman rocking violently back and forth in his chair; another one bangs again and again on a plastic garbage can; a madwoman cackles at some joke only she can hear; and there's a brief confrontation when one brushes against another—why are you touching me? Why Are You Touching Me!? Then there are those with some settled calm, weary with the weight of medication, yet present and trying to surface, trying to understand the newness being forced on them. And finally, there are those who have found their own power, their own voices, brilliant against the prevalent greys, as if colour was splashed where none was allowed before—as if Ted Turner had colourized black-and-white movies. A hospital administrator at the gathering says to me in mistaken pride, "You know, they didn't want to go." They didn't want to leave rehab and their workers there to go to a survivor business; they didn't want to make this move away from the passive to the empowered. Of course, they didn't; dependence is the hallmark of institutional care. For the community of psychiatric survivors, and even for the staff, however, there has to be a way for change. We need to look at our very negative experiences in a way that can help us shed the guilt, the shame, and failure.

Not so long ago, there was no colour at all. Coming into the hospital then was like walking into bedlam—it was not a place of hope or of high expectation. The building confined us, after we had been culled from the main population—that living, working, striving population that still participated in the race for success. We all took on the same pallor, the same slump in the shoulders, the same shuffling gait. We took on as well the behaviours that we saw around us and we learned a new language to express all the pain, grief, and loss. Illness became the major feature of our lives; it became the only thing that brought us those precious moments of attention from exasperated staff—and that attention was the only break in the silent sameness of the days.

Decades ago, they used to keep those labelled mentally ill in bed. Nurses in starched white uniforms watched over dormitory-sized wards, and moved from patient to patient distributing medications, as though rest and inactivity were all that was needed to return people to a semblance of health. The uniforms and dormitory wards are gone now, but hospital staff still discourage expectations, movement, and hope; they push acceptance of our limitations, our illnesses, and our empty lives.

A couple of days from now, survivors will hold a workshop here, funded by a grant to Accent on Ability, the charitable foundation created by Away Express Couriers. We will talk about the survivor movement and address some of the fears and concerns of this reluctant new membership. We will encourage and cajole. I watch the faces around me and wonder what words will reach them.

         ·   ·   ·

By the time Laurie Hall and I arrived for the workshop at the hospital, people were already gathering for the meeting. Some sat chatting in the room and others collected at the entrance, dragging the last puffs from their smokes. Getting survivors out to meetings is always tricky—once home, there is a reluctance to venture out. No matter how bad the physical space inside, it's safer than outside. And the effects of medications leave people tired and unmotivated; it's difficult to concentrate or to sit still for any period of time.

On the drive to the hospital, Laurie Hall and I decided that she would speak after me and that we'd keep our talks short, punchy, and upbeat. For more than a decade, Laurie had been the highly respected executive director of Away Express Couriers. She had been a hero to her staff, and in the broader movement she was a woman who symbolized our fledgling ambitions to raise ourselves up and grab hold of life. A compact, attractive woman with an easy smile and a throaty laugh, Laurie has deep, self-inflicted scars covering her arms. These road maps of her pain are at odds with the confidence, humour, and quiet charisma that she exudes.

We understood the new OTW staff were suspicious of activists like us. Perhaps they feared that they would be persuaded to hate their workers, or to stop taking their medications, or to deny that mental illness even existed. Part of this misapprehension came from the staff and part of it from themselves.

Neither Laurie nor I expected the high turnout, although our intention was to have as many survivor role models as possible show up. Barry D'Costa, the intense and popular director of Parkdale's Green Thumb Enterprises, was there and had brought his staff along to sit with the Out of This World Café folks. The Raging Spoon was doing the catering, and Away staff were also present.

As I prepared to speak, I thought about the ghosts I live with—from my former boarding home and from the Parkdale drop-in where I worked for seven years with "chronic mental patients." They had died without hope, without recognition of their worth, and without acknowledgment of their potential. It seemed to me that these ghosts were gathering here, in this unlikely place, leaning against the walls, watching with a mixture of approval and sadness as we tried to reach this audience of the still living, still breathing. Those ghosts are my touchstones, my motivation, and they are never far from me.

I started off the session:

"Almost twenty-five years ago, I was sent to Channan Court in Parkdale to live out my life. Someone had decided I was a chronic mental patient, and the best thing, maybe the only thing, for me was to be in a place where I would be taken care of, a supervised environment where my meals would be prepared for me, and my room and board paid by a grudging government.

"There were seventy people in the house, mostly men, from Whitby and the Lakeshore and Queen Street. The rooms were crowded and dirty, the meals the cheapest possible and the days terribly long and despairing. There was little for people to do, nothing to wake up for, except to grab coffee and cereal before it ran out, and then return to bed.

"It felt like we'd been given up on, and so it was natural that we mostly gave up on ourselves.

"We didn't like to risk going outside—people would stare, children would tease—so we stayed in, and our bodies got soft and flabby from lack of exercise and from food that was mostly starch: bread, potatoes, and spaghetti. Our minds got dull too, with nothing to spark thought or real conversation as our world shrunk inside the walls of the boarding home.

"There were very few visitors, and it was very hard to tell the days apart—only cheque day stood out, and that was over so fast and took so long to come again it hardly counted. Though we never really talked about how we felt, living the way we were, if it could be called living, there was a great deal of sadness in the house. We knew our lives were fading out, that we'd never really had a chance to do the things that make life worth living—finding work that we could enjoy, finding a partner to love and grow with, having a real home. So we felt bad, but we thought that feeling that was just part of our mental illness, something that only medication could control. No one said to us: Of course you feel terrible, how could you not, living here? Of course you feel sad, look at what you've been denied!

"And because we did nothing, because there was nothing to do, workers thought we could do nothing more, and that it might be dangerous to expect anything else from us other than simply existing.

"We were wrong, and they were wrong.

"But it took us a long, long time to be able to say that, to mean that, to show that. First we had to show ourselves, and that was very scary. It meant risking again, trying again, daring to hope that things might be better for us. As bad as things were in the boarding and rooming houses, it was the devil we knew, and the thought of leaving that, for me, was very frightening. Change for us never meant anything great; it usually came in increases in rent and the cost of cigarettes, and in cutbacks in our cheques. We

don't trust change. And we don't trust ourselves. Our bodies are so
exhausted, so unused to movement, partly from the medications,
partly from lousy diets, partly from a realistic depression that saps
any strength right out of our bones. And sometimes its hard to
kick-start our brains, they feel shrouded in fog, sluggish and slow—
and though we think that is from the illness, mostly it's from the
rusting over that happens when there is nothing in our environment, in our surroundings, to stimulate thought and reason.

"Because we're poor, because we are constantly struggling just
to keep food in our bellies and a roof, any roof, over our heads,
there's been little room for anything else in these lives we lead. If
we look to communities where the poor live, in Metro housing
projects, for example, we can see how destructive simple poverty
can be. How fear and want rule those communities, along with
shame and despair.

"We're poor. And we have, on top of that poverty, a mental illness. A double whammy. We are more than whatever mental
illness afflicts us, but sometimes we forget that, and the system
we're in forgets that, and the government forgets that.

"Over the last few decades, our struggle has been fought on a
number of different fronts, by some people whose names you
know and others you may not have heard of—to increase our
rights to participate in decision-making within the hospital,
to ensure our rights are known and protected, to create better
housing; and though we may not have fully understood where
we were going with all that activity, we know now that we were,
we are, fighting for the right to be seen as whole individuals, as

people rather than as diseases, individuals who are entitled to opportunities, to work and to learn and to fulfill their potential. We are in the business of human development.

"This is not wide-eyed radicalism; this is not a group of people who will tell you to flush your medications down the toilet, or hate your therapist, or never be admitted to hospital again. These are people, and I'm one of them, who've lived with the same feelings you've endured, and who've been out in the world looking around, testing the water, and finding things out. These are some of the things we've learned:

"We've found out that, like in the movie *What About Bob?* it's about taking little steps, finding the emotional wherewithal and courage to try again. You've already taken that first step by signing up in a survivor business.

"We've found out that there are other, better ways to live, that we can grab on to, that are achievable.

"We've found out that we are quite capable of learning, of growing, of mining our human potential. Some of us may learn differently than others, but that just means we have to find the best ways to teach—one size does not fit all.

"We've found out that poverty is de-humanizing, terribly limiting, and leaves little room for hope.

"We've found out how much strength we really have, to still be walking, talking, and breathing. So we call ourselves psychiatric survivors, turning shame into pride.

"We found that unless we use our bodies, they grow soft and take much more energy to move.

"We found that unless we challenge our minds, they grow dull.

"We found that our community needs role models, leaders, to give us hope, to show what we can achieve.

"We found that much of what we thought was part and parcel of our mental illness was in fact grief and loss and loneliness and fear.

"We found we can grow bigger than this illness, and it will shrink like a tumour under chemotherapy as we nourish ourselves with expectations and accomplishments, with friends who are also struggling to break out of the passive, institutional role, as we find reasons to get out of bed in the mornings and reasons to sleep well at night.

"We found support where we least expected it, in government and in agencies like Trillium and United Way, in people like former mayor Barbara Hall, in academics and even in communities that used to reject us.

"We'd like you to find all that too."

Laurie understands the effect she has on people, whether they're bureaucrats or survivors; she also knows the burdens and obligations of leadership. She's come a long way in a short time—from being a frequent psychiatric hospital patient to being a leader who can help others find their own paths. With her trademark casual approach, she grabs the attention of the audience, peppering her talk with irreverent remarks about being a "mental case." She talks about her repeated hospital admissions, suicide attempts, and her life on the street. She then tells how coming across Away Express saved her life, giving her back the sense of community that had been stolen from her; how what had seemed beyond her (showing up for shifts on those days when the turmoil in her head told her to stay in bed) became easy after a while; how she advanced to office work and learned computer skills; how she gathered up the courage to apply for the executive director job when it became available, and her shock at getting it.

We asked the workshop participants to talk about their own ambitions and to say what they'd thought about being before they were labelled, and then set aside. And they did, beginning with someone from the Out of This World staff who tentatively put up her hand and said she'd wanted to be a nurse. The floodgates opened as fifty people—scarred by hardscrabble lives—sat for three hours, remarkable in itself, hungrily paying profound attention to the speakers and each other. There was so much emotion in the room, and no one to bring us medications to ward off these unaccustomed feelings. Here we were in the very belly of the beast.

Louis talked of starting out washing dishes in the Spoon, and how he'd moved up to doing office work for OCAB.

"It's about independence," he declared. "Being able to afford your own apartment."

A PERC member talked about discovering her own hidden talents as she worked on bidding contracts; another wanted to learn to write; a young woman talked about creating community gardens so that the poor could have access to fresh vegetables;

people congratulated and thanked one another. Pat Fowler talked about travelling to England, Scotland, and Ireland with a documentary called *Working Like Crazy* that OCAB had participated in, which gave a profile of her and others. She spoke about how well survivors there had received them: "They're just like us. They laugh at the same things, and they worry about the same things."

Barry D'Costa was emotional as he welcomed his "brothers and sisters" at the OTW, pledging to help any way he could. He affirmed that they were now part of a large and growing community of survivors who were breaking stereotypes and caring for one another.

Nobody wanted to leave.

The highlight came when the coordinator of OTW announced with excitement and pride that their staff now had keys giving them access to all the wards. Nothing spoke so clearly of change as this—it was our own Bastille Day.

Epilogue

Most of us simply don't want to hurt anymore.

Our pain makes us soft targets for pharmaceuticals, and not-so-legal drugs, to smooth the jagged edges of our feelings and make the unbearable bearable. We must realize, however, that as chaotic and dangerous as the world sometimes seems, it's the only one we've got, and we must face it. Turning our back on it by taking drugs or reducing it to the house we live in or the street we glimpse from our window will bring great sadness. We need to plug back in to society, whether it wants us to or not. We need to go to work on ourselves and on our community. We need to help make things better for others, and this will transform our own lives in ways we never expected.

None of us knows our own potential, and we never will unless we strive to fulfill it. I know with certainty that we are not here to seek revenge on parents or on the world that failed us. And if there is an afterlife that demands an account of ourselves, a note from a psychiatrist won't be much help.

Years ago, when Laurie Hall was dying (by her own hand) on her hospital bed, she would never have believed that what lay before her was everything she was searching for: love, acceptance, work, and respect. She had to reach a point where she could draw on her strengths, face her nightmare, and move on. When she was ready, Away Express was there for her as a first stepping-stone to all that she would become. Now she stands shoulder to shoulder with other survivor activists, and she has learned to laugh and to let the pain recede on most days. She is valued, and every day people let her know that.

Barry D'Costa, too, has found a firm place to stand and a way to give. He works with his Green Thumb Enterprises crew (drawn from members of the Parc drop-in) to carry out their contracts with the local business associations planting, watering, and maintaining flowers and small trees in the cement planters that dot the neighbourhoods of Queen Street West and Roncesvalles. Watching him, it is easy to see that he has transformed his pain into empathy and determination. He is a caring person who is much loved. Surrounded by affection, he no longer has to stand powerless in the face of suffering.

Jill Stainsby is going for her MA in social work, partly for her own edification and partly to keep her job in the new political regime of British Columbia that has borrowed Mike Harris's hatchet and is wielding it against social services. At the same time, she organizes gay square dancing, takes care of her cats and her tidy apartment, and teaches others respectful ways to encourage members of our community to break out of lethargy and drug-induced comas.

Lee Robson continues her work, helping people at their lowest point understand—simply by her mere presence—that it is possible to break out of the cycle of illness and hospitalization, and find meaningful work for real pay. She continues with her crafts, sharing her skills and her products, while her mother's ghost plays less and less of a role in her life.

Julie Flatt just keeps getting stronger, growing, and taking on new responsibilities. She and Laurie are working together now at the revamped Ontario Peer Development Initiative. Talk about dream teams.

Carol Janzen feels great these days; her home life is better, and she will get her degree. She has found a medication that lets her live and study and feel some of the good that's out there. She can nourish and love her children and accept herself.

Allan Strong loves his children, his wife, his community, his work, and his life. His group in Kitchener-Waterloo emphasizes wellness, not sickness, and he still laughs that laugh I know so well.

Young Cheryl Gray won a partial scholarship from Children's Aid and started at the University of Toronto this past fall. Her father is so proud of her that he sometimes cries when he looks at her, but they are now tears of joy. She and Barry are members of the FMP Collective (we're all Former Mental Patients), our writing group that plans to publish an anthology of survivor writing from across Canada. She is thrilled to have been asked to serve on the board of the Gerstein Centre.

Pat Fowler continues her work with Diana at OCAB, her own transformation still a source of much pride for everyone around her. A very competent, loving, attractive woman, Pat is far removed from the "freak" she once felt herself to be.

Dan Carter has no time for self-pity or liquid escapes. He's taken on another television show as well as the one he already

does, and he has expanded his viewing audience. He does a
remarkable amount of public speaking, and is always inspira-
tional. Who can tell the number of lives that may have changed
because of him?

Diana Capponi travels throughout Ontario to small towns
and remote regions carrying messages of hope and encourage-
ment to isolated pockets of survivors: What we have done, you
can do too; step towards life, not away from it, the rewards are
profound. Everywhere she goes, she leaves behind a determined
group that is ready to use the tools she has given them to build a
business, to build a life.

As for me, on most days I'm filled with a deep sense of pride
and shared accomplishment. We are survivors, and more than
just survivors: we are groundbreakers and role models and teachers and leaders. And though there remains much to do, much to
fight, much to plan, we have made a tremendous start, for
ourselves and for others.

Madness will never be the same.

Index